The Little Book
of
CBD
for
Self-Care

The Little Book
of
CBD
for
Self-Care

175+ Ways to Soothe, Support,
& Restore Yourself with CBD

Sophie Saint Thomas

Adams Media
New York London Toronto Sydney New Delhi

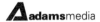

Adams Media
An Imprint of Simon & Schuster, Inc.
57 Littlefield Street
Avon, Massachusetts 02322

First Adams Media hardcover edition September 2020

ADAMS MEDIA and colophon are trademarks of Simon & Schuster.

For information about special discounts for bulk purchases, please contact Simon & Schuster Special Sales at 1-866-506-1949 or business@simonandschuster.com.

The Simon & Schuster Speakers Bureau can bring authors to your live event. For more information or to book an event contact the Simon & Schuster Speakers Bureau at 1-866-248-3049 or visit our website at www.simonspeakers.com.

Interior design by Colleen Cunningham
Images © 123RF/Pavel Lunevich

Manufactured in the United States of America

10 9 8 7 6 5 4 3 2 1

Library of Congress Cataloging-in-Publication Data
Names: Saint Thomas, Sophie, author.
Title: The little book of CBD for self-care / Sophie Saint Thomas.
Description: Avon, Massachusetts: Adams Media, 2020. | Includes bibliographical references.
Identifiers: LCCN 2020011314 | ISBN 9781507213636 (hc) | ISBN 9781507213643 (ebook)
Subjects: LCSH: Cannabinoids--Therapeutic use--Popular works. | Cannabinoids--Health aspects--Popular works. | Self-care, Health--Popular works.
Classification: LCC RM666.C266 S254 2020 | DDC 615.7/827--dc23
LC record available at https://lccn.loc.gov/2020011314

ISBN 978-1-5072-1363-6
ISBN 978-1-5072-1364-3 (ebook)

Contents

Self-Care Exercises

Introduction

You work hard. You take care of your friends, family, and partner. Whatever you're doing, you give it your all. But when you're so busy making sure that everyone else is happy, it's easy to forget that you need rest and care too. Fortunately, CBD can help you slow down, relax, improve your overall sense of well-being, and more. It can also be used to elevate your approach to self-care, and that's where *The Little Book of CBD for Self-Care* comes in.

Self-care is the practice of slowing down and taking steps to put yourself first. It is the simple understanding that you deserve love, and the realization that if you are happy, so are those around you. In today's busy world, taking a break to do something you love without shame or guilt takes courage. But here you'll find more than 175 CBD-enhanced self-care activities that will help you rejuvenate your mind, body, and spirit, along with a section that teaches you more about CBD and the impact it can have on your self-care practice. So turn the page and get ready to prioritize yourself for a change.

CBD and Self-Care

CBD helps you relax. This plant molecule may be calming, but it's not weak. It goes to battle against the anxious and ruminating thoughts that stand between you and self-care. After CBD opens the door for tranquility, it provides an array of self-soothing benefits, from pain relief to stress reduction. Let's explore how to utilize it to maximize your potential.

What Is Self-Care?

Self-care is treating yourself the way you would treat other people. It means listening to yourself and taking care of your needs. It is what you do to prioritize *you*—mind, body, and spirit.

In today's hectic society, steeped in social media and a 24/7 news cycle, there is pressure to go, go, go. However, if you don't take a break and integrate self-care into your life—whether once a day, once a week, or more often—you risk health problems and burnout. Treating yourself well isn't frivolous; it's crucial to surviving in this tough world. Your body needs enough sleep, water, and exercise. Your mind needs stimulation. And your spirit needs love. Self-care honors life by striving to make yours as happy and healthy as possible.

The way that you practice self-care is up to you. A luxurious bath may be perfect for one person; someone else may need a day spent working hard in the garden. But whatever you need, you'll find what you're looking for in this book. Self-care is self-love, so let's take a look at the different types of self-care and how CBD can help you connect with and nurture the whole you.

Body

Your body is the vessel that carries you through this life. With the aid of CBD, physical self-care can alleviate pain and help you feel more comfortable. Then you can focus on what your body both wants and needs, such as exercise, massage, or more sleep. When your body is happy and running smoothly, the rest of life falls more easily into place.

Mind

In a world filled with constant news and social media posts, it's easy to feel stressed out. Fortunately, by practicing mental self-care you can curate the content of your mind, creating a paradise where stress is only welcome when useful.

Mental self-care will help you take care of tasks and chores and enjoy yourself while you do so. And if it's hard to turn off your mind and focus inward, you'll find meditations, breath work, and more throughout these pages that will teach you to quiet your mind and sink into total relaxation. Using CBD to enhance your mental self-care will help you relax, have fun, and focus on what makes you happy.

Spirit

Your spirit is you in your true form. It's the joy you feel from baking brownies for a loved one, playing with your pet, or going on an adventure all by yourself. CBD helps lower your stress levels and empty your mind of the negative thoughts that hold you back so you can be mindful, joyous, and free in the present moment.

What Is CBD?

Cannabidiol, or CBD, is a phytocannabinoid, a chemical plant compound that occurs naturally in plants in the cannabis family. Both the marijuana plant, which contains the psychoactive chemical compound tetrahydrocannabinol (THC), and the hemp plant, which most CBD is currently derived from, are part of this family. Hemp contains 0.3 percent or less of THC, which isn't enough to produce a psychoactive effect.

While a lot more research still needs to be done on CBD, what researchers know so far is that when CBD enters the body, it binds with receptors in the endocannabinoid system (ECS). Your ECS is an internal biological system that is believed to play a crucial role in maintaining homeostasis, your body's ability to maintain a state of internal balance and well-being regardless of changes and outside factors. Within the ECS, there are two primary cannabinoid receptors: CB1 and CB2. CB1 receptors are the most abundant in the brain and are the ones that THC interacts with to produce a high. CB2 receptors exist mostly in the immune system. Currently, researchers don't know exactly how CBD interacts with the ECS, but they do know that it doesn't bind to CB1 or CB2 receptors in the same way THC does. One popular theory is that CBD works by preventing endocannabinoids from being broken down. This means they can have a greater effect on your body. Other researchers propose that CBD may bind to a receptor that hasn't yet been discovered.

Again, while THC is psychoactive, CBD won't get you high. Instead, CBD can do everything from making your skin glow to restoring calm to fighting pain. CBD helps you be your best self without risk of dependence, which makes it perfect for self-care. Let's take a closer look at how CBD can help you prioritize your mind, body, and spirit.

What Can CBD Do?

Right now, most of the research on CBD concerns its anti-inflammatory and anti-anxiety effects, but these two sides of CBD allow for a number of supplementary benefits that you can use to enhance your self-care practice. CBD can soothe pain, care for your skin, and make you feel more comfortable in your body, all important aspects of physical self-care. It can also help you relax, de-stress, practice mindfulness, and push away your worries, all of which are crucial for mental and spiritual self-care.

Let's take a closer look at the benefits of CBD.

Reduces Inflammation and Pain

Inflammation helps your body fight off infection, but too much inflammation leads to weight gain and disease. By connecting with certain receptor sites in your body, cannabidiol reduces inflammation, treating everything from headaches, hangovers, and muscle soreness to puffy eyes, chronic pain, and epilepsy, as suggested in a 2018 study published in *Surgical Neurology International*. By both relieving and preventing common ailments and discomforts, CBD's anti-inflammatory properties make it easier to settle into the present and focus on self-care.

Nourishes Skin and Hair

CBD is rapidly becoming popular for its role in beauty and skin care. A 2013 study published in the *British Journal of Clinical Pharmacology* suggests that CBD can increase blood flow, which explains its beauty benefits. Blood flow helps by balancing sebum (oil) production, keeping pores clean. This encourages hair growth and collagen production while also reducing acne and signs of aging. The phytocannabinoid anti-inflammatory properties can also nourish the scalp, treat acne, combat dryness, and leave you feeling strong and looking fresh and renewed. Researchers also found that CBD can prevent acne from forming in the first place by preventing cells from producing excess oil. Additionally, a 2019 study found that the cannabinoid helps the skin by regulating its homeostasis. CBD's magic is its ability to make you both look and feel good through the same mechanisms.

Boosts Mood and Decreases Stress

A 2019 study showed how CBD acts on the brain's receptors for serotonin, which regulates your mood and can help decrease anxiety, stress, and depression. Additional research shows that CBD can also lower your fear response. When you're able to decrease the potency of these uncomfortable emotions (fear, stress, etc.), you are able to be more fully present in your own life. You're able to take care of yourself and feel more comfortable and confident in your body.

By lowering anxiety and your stress response, CBD can also help you sink into relaxation—whether you're coming down with a cold or just in need of some rest. The cannabinoid can also help you let your guard down and open up emotionally, aiding in intimacy with friends, family, and partners.

Helps You Get Motivated, Creative, and Focused

It's difficult to get anything done with anxious and ruminating thoughts. While more research still needs to be done on CBD's direct ability to increase focus, CBD enthusiasts across the country report using the compound to brainstorm, stay in the moment, and get motivated. This is likely due to CBD's anxiety-relieving properties. When you brush away those distractions, you can focus on the task at hand much more easily and brush away creative blocks. Additionally, feeling productive can help boost your self-esteem, and canceling out any stress-induced thoughts allows you to fully immerse yourself in soothing and joyful activities, like the self-care activities found throughout this book.

Treats Nausea, Stimulates Appetite, and Boosts Metabolism

A 2011 study published in the *British Journal of Pharmacology* found that CBD can relieve nausea and vomiting, and researchers also believe the compound can stimulate appetite. Busy schedules and everyday stress can lead to uncomfortable GI issues or may cause you to skip meals. CBD can help you remember to take care of these basic needs so you can operate at full capacity—and enjoy some delicious and healthy foods! Additionally, early research suggests that CBD can boost metabolism by interacting with lymphoid tissue and the brain, helping to regulate a healthy appetite.

Helps with Insomnia and Encourages Sleep

CBD can help alleviate insomnia and help you get a good night's sleep. As we've discussed, CBD can be fantastic for lowering stress, anxiety, worries, and pain—all of which are most likely the things that keep you up at night. One 2019 study found that 79 percent of the patients treated with CBD reported lower anxiety levels and 67 percent slept better.

Sleep deprivation can lead to irritability, anxiety, mood swings, and reduction in your productivity at home and at work. It's also harder to enjoy everyday life and your friends and family when you're exhausted. CBD is a natural sleep aid that can help you avoid these things. Most clinical trials on CBD and sleep gave subjects 25–1,500 milligrams of CBD, so start with small doses and speak with your doctor to determine what works best for you.

Works As a Nutritional Supplement

Because it comes from a plant, CBD can work as a nutritional supplement. Early research suggests that CBD has antibiotic properties. While you shouldn't skip traditional antibiotics the next time you need them, CBD's antibiotic properties add extra incentive to incorporate it into your regimen. You can add CBD and hemp oil, seeds, and even leaves to everything from savory dishes to smoothies.

Full Spectrum, Broad Spectrum, and Isolate

Now that you know how CBD can help enhance your self-care, you need to know what to buy. When browsing CBD products, you will notice the terms *full spectrum*, *broad spectrum*, and *isolate*. These three different products refer to the method by which the CBD is extracted from the plant and the plant's cannabinoid profile.

Let's take a look at each type.

Full Spectrum

Full-spectrum CBD, also referred to as "whole plant" CBD, extracts the cannabinoid CBD and everything else with it, including the plant's terpenes (additional compounds responsible for taste, smell, and even calming benefits). Since CBD is made from a plant with less than 0.3 percent of THC, you don't need to worry about psychoactive effects. Some people prefer full spectrum because it's said to contain more nutrients. The "entourage effect" refers to the belief that CBD works best when you keep all its friends (other plant compounds) with it.

Broad Spectrum

Broad-spectrum CBD contains most, but not all, of the other plant compounds that come with CBD. Some people prefer to avoid any THC, even nonpsychoactive levels. Broad spectrum uses a refinement process that removes all the THC (and as a result, some of the other plant compounds), while leaving in all the CBD and most of the other good stuff.

Isolate

CBD isolate is just that: isolated CBD. It's gone through more rigorous extraction processes to ensure that your product is pure CBD and nothing but CBD. Compared to the natural brown or yellow of full-spectrum and broad-spectrum products, CBD isolate is usually pure white.

Intake Methods and Dosing

How should you consume your CBD? There are a few options with various onset times, benefits, and uses. Try one or all of these CBD intake methods. Remember, CBD is safe and nonpsychoactive, so it's okay to explore to find the right dose for you.

CBD dosing depends on a few things, such as body weight, pain level, your unique body chemistry, and the method of intake. A good rule of thumb is to take 1–6 milligrams of CBD for every 10 pounds of body weight with respect to your pain needs. Following that formula, 20 milligrams is a safe starting dose for everyone. So start with 20 milligrams, add as needed, and keep a journal of your experience.

* **Sublingual Tincture:** A sublingual tincture is CBD suspended in alcohol that you can place under your tongue or add to your favorite beverage. Start with 20 milligrams a day, or about 4 drops, increasing the dose as needed. CBD is available in a variety of strengths. For instance, in a 500 milligram strength, a 1 milliliter dropper contains 16 milligrams of CBD; but a 1,000 milligram strength yields twice that. For

the purposes of this book, we'll assume you're using a 500 milligram–strength tincture, available in a 30 milliliter bottle. Sublingual tinctures last a long time and come in discreet and often beautiful bottles. They kick in 15–45 minutes after consumption and last for 2–3 hours, so they are helpful to combine with self-care activities that combat stress.

* **Oil:** Often oil, such as coconut oil or olive oil, is used in a CBD tincture rather than alcohol. CBD oil can be added to many recipes, from facial masks to multi-course dinners. Start with 20 milligrams a day, or about 4 drops, increasing your dose as needed. Like with an alcohol-based tincture, you'll feel the effects 15–45 minutes after consuming it, and it will last for 2–3 hours. CBD oil is great for stress relief or any self-care activity that requires near-immediate effects.

* **Topical:** A CBD topical is a lotion, cream, or oil that is applied directly to the skin. While other intake methods offer overall pain relief, a topical works directly on the area of discomfort. Topicals take roughly 1 hour to kick in and can last for up to 6 hours. While there is no standard dosage for topicals, as it varies person to person, try starting with 7.5 milliliters to get a 30 milligram dose of CBD and apply more to the region as needed. Use CBD topicals for self-care activities involving skin care and localized pain relief.

* **Powder:** Some companies sell CBD isolate in powdered form. It's easy to add CBD powder to smoothies or even dissolve it in water as a beverage. Powders take about 1 hour to become effective and last 6–8 hours.

* **Edibles:** *Edible* is an umbrella term that refers to any CBD that you eat. This means CBD gummies made with oil, brownies made with high-CBD hemp plant or capsules, and more. The exact dosage and onset time of edibles vary, but you can begin with roughly 20 milligrams of CBD per serving. Allow at least 1 hour for the compound to take effect. Results should last for 6–8 hours, making edibles perfect for self-care activities that last an entire day, afternoon, or night out.

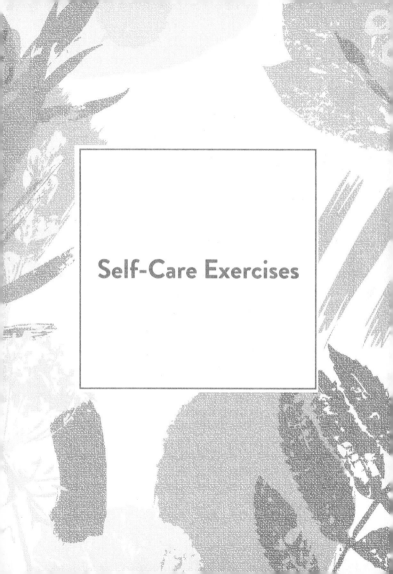

Self-Care Exercises

Stretch It Out

How does it help?

Stretching enhances relaxation while improving posture and range of motion and reducing muscle stiffness. Massaging some CBD on your muscles prestretch can help make these benefits even better. If you are sore afterward, CBD can help heal muscles by fighting inflammation.

How to:

1. Sit on a yoga mat with your legs straight out in front of you. Have a CBD topical by your side.
2. Slowly, vertebra by vertebra, recline back onto your yoga mat until you are lying down. Notice your back elongating. Point your toes and wiggle them. Raise your hands above your head and reach for the back wall, making your body as long as you can. Hold this pose for 10–12 breaths.
3. Place your hands back by your side. Mentally scan your body for aches and soreness, then gently, vertebra by vertebra, sit back up. Using circular motions, rub the CBD topical into any area of your body that's sore.
4. Now gently, on your yoga mat, slowly enter a stretch your body is craving. Once you're finished, apply more topical to any lingering sore areas.

Turn Your Bed Into a Temple

How does it help?

Creating an environment conducive to rest helps you fall asleep, so let CBD help you focus on and create your dream bed. Then sleep through the night in your comfy new setup by taking CBD before bedtime.

How to:

1. Take CBD to enter a calm, focused headspace. Grab a pen and journal and draw your dream sleep setup. Perhaps it's the sound of crashing waves and the tranquil color blue. Maybe romantic red roses on the bedside table appeals to you.

2. Settle into CBD relaxation. Download white noise apps on your phone. Replace your sheets. What about an eye mask and some calming lavender oil on your bedside table? Create your dream bed—you deserve it!

3. Research shows that CBD promotes restful sleep and treats insomnia. Keep some by your bedside table. Take a few capsules or tincture drops and snuggle into your slumber paradise.

Give Yourself a Scalp Massage

How does it help?

Taking care of your scalp is crucial for healthy hair. A scalp massage stimulates circulation to the hair follicles, which promotes hair growth. Additionally, a CBD scalp massage increases your brain's levels of serotonin—the "happy" chemical—making this self-care activity one that will leave you feeling good inside and out.

How to:

1. Place several drops of CBD-infused oil into the palm of your hands, then rub them together to warm up the oil.
2. Start at the front of your scalp and gently rub in circular motions. Practice deep breathing as you work.
3. Being careful not to tangle your hair, slowly and methodically move toward the back of the head.
4. Continue until you've massaged your whole head and feel relaxed and happy.

Make a Green Tea Mockito

How does it help?

CBD acts as a healthy alcohol alternative that relaxes you without the risk of a hangover. Practice self-care by staying social at events and sipping a drink that facilitates calm and stops social stress.

You will need:

5 mint leaves, 1 tablespoon lime juice, CBD sugar to taste (or regular sugar plus 20 milligrams CBD tincture), ice, 2 ounces brewed green tea (cooled), sparkling water to fill

How to:

1. In a tall glass, muddle 4 mint leaves, lime juice, and CBD sugar (or sugar with CBD tincture added). The mint leaves should bruise. Let them sit for a few minutes so the flavors can marry.
2. Add ice ⅔ of the way to the top of the glass. Pour green tea on top.
3. Pour sparkling water to fill the glass all the way to the top. Garnish with the last mint leaf and enjoy.

Play with Your Pets

How does it help?

Get silly with your furry friends! Playing with your pets increases your connection with them while providing an instant mood boost. Studies suggest that CBD interacts with the brain in a way that reduces stress, which will allow you to practice this self-care activity by letting go and really feeling playful and free.

How to:

1. Take CBD by your preferred method, whether in a tincture, capsules, or other form. Then hang out with your pet for a few minutes.
2. Once you're feeling calm and happy from the CBD, start playing. Give your pet snuggles, play tag, build a pillow fort, go to the dog park. Let your pet run the show as an act of mindfulness.
3. When you're done playing, reflect on what you learned. Does your pet truly dance like no one is watching? Do they show unbridled affection? Animals can teach you a lot about your human hang-ups to help you become your best version of yourself.

Take Polaroids

How does it help?

A Polaroid photo shoot is an analog way to have fun and capture memories—no screen time required. Having a hard time relaxing? Sometimes being the center of attention can be tough. Take a CBD tincture, which kicks in after 15–45 minutes, then enjoy your self-care photo shoot with a friend.

How to:

1. Next time you get together with a friend, bring your CBD tincture and a Polaroid camera. Enjoy CBD (with your friend's consent, of course). Watch how it gently lowers your inhibitions, calms nerves, and helps you open up to each other emotionally.
2. Take out your Polaroid camera. With Polaroids, there's no risk of posting or sharing, of liking or not liking. It's just a tangible memory.
3. Do your best fashion model impression and take photos until you run out of film.
4. Sip more calming CBD beverages as you watch the photos develop. Give them to your friend, put them in a scrapbook, or tuck them away somewhere for safekeeping.

Lift Weights

How does it help?

Lifting weights can help you lose fat, increase muscle tone, and improve your bone density while making you stronger and more confident. But as your muscles develop, you may feel some aches and pains. Adding CBD to your weight lifting routine eases sore muscles, so you only need to focus on your workout.

How to:

1. Take CBD in a capsule or tincture each morning as a supplement to fight inflammation and get ahead of muscle pain before it starts.
2. Head to the gym and start lifting. Enjoy the feeling of doing something solely for yourself as you practice this self-care activity. If you're not sure how to start, see if your gym offers a free personal training session.
3. Listen to your body. If you feel pain, stop. Only use weights that you can lift 12–15 times comfortably in a row. Form is important, so work at a rate and weight that allows you to maintain good form.

Practice Abdominal Breathing

How does it help?

Relieving stress reduces irritability, can increase your intuition, improves memory, and boosts physical health. Ease your stress by trying abdominal breathing, which increases the flow of oxygen to your body and reduces physical tension. Couple this self-care exercise with CBD's stress-busting powers for maximum relief.

How to:

1. Sit in a comfortable position on your yoga mat or a pillow. Ingest some CBD, relax, and feel the day's anxiety begin to lessen in your body. You carry stress that can manifest as physical aches and pains.
2. Place one hand on your belly and the other on your chest.
3. Take a deep breath in through your nose. Watch your belly push your hand out. Keep your chest still.
4. Breathe out deeply through pursed lips as if you were whistling. The hand on your belly will sink back in. Use your hand to push all the air out. Feel the tension you carry in your chest and shoulders release with your exhale.
5. Repeat 10 times. If you'd like, bookend your practice by consuming CBD after you're finished. Note how your body feels more comfortable and relaxed.

Make and Use a CBD Bath Bomb

How does it help?

Making a CBD bath bomb is a playful and productive act of mindfulness. Then you can relieve stress, aches, and pains by plopping it in the bath. Bath bombs are a great way to apply a topical to your entire body.

You will need:

Latex gloves, 1 cup baking soda, ½ cup citric acid, ½ cup Epsom salts, ½ cup cornstarch, 2 tablespoons warm/room-temperature coconut oil (you just don't want it to be solid), 1 teaspoon water, 2–3 drops green food coloring, 1,000 milligrams CBD oil, bath bomb mold or muffin tin

How to:

1. Put on your gloves, then combine baking soda, citric acid, Epsom salts, and cornstarch in a large bowl.
2. In a separate bowl, combine coconut oil, water, food coloring, and CBD oil.
3. Slowly pour the wet mixture into the dry mixture, whisking continuously. The consistency should be like crumbly sand. Once mixed, tightly pack the mixture into a bath bomb mold or muffin tin and let it set overnight.
4. Gently remove the bath bomb from the mold and crack it open, then draw a bath. Drop the bath bomb into the tub and relax with CBD.

Recover from a Cold

How does it help?

Did you know that stress can lead to colds? Manage stress with CBD. If you're already feeling run-down, practice self-care by using CBD to rest and get back to full functionality.

How to:

1. When you begin feeling under the weather, allow yourself to rest. Consume some CBD to relax.

2. Use a full-spectrum CBD product. Hemp, which most CBD is made from, contains vitamin C, zinc, and protein to help you feel better. While CBD helps you sink into your couch and sleep, it also reduces cold-related aches and pains and helps your body heal.

3. Drink lots of fluids. Add a few drops of CBD tincture to your water to flush out the toxins. Stay tuned in to your body and use CBD as long as you need to rest up so you can return to your full strength. Honoring your body and allowing it to rest will help you get better faster so you can return to your busy routine.

Try CBD Honey

How does it help?

Following a recipe is science. It stimulates your mind while acting as a mindfulness activity by forcing you to focus on the step-by-step instructions. This healing, delicious self-care activity lets you double up on honey's anti-inflammatory properties by adding CBD.

You will need:

2-cup glass measuring cup, candy thermometer, 1,000 milligrams CBD tincture, 2 cups honey

How to:

1. Create a double boiler by filling a small saucepan with water and placing the glass measuring cup inside. Set the saucepan on medium heat and heat the water to 95°F, using the thermometer to ensure the temperature doesn't get too high. If the water gets too hot, you risk burning away the antibacterial benefits of the honey.
2. Pour CBD tincture into the glass measuring cup, then add honey.
3. Stir the product until it's at a consistency you enjoy. Remove the glass measuring cup from the heat and cool.
4. Eat a spoonful of honey, close your eyes, relax, and focus on you as you try this sweet, antibiotic, and anti-inflammatory treat.

Put Together an On-the-Go CBD Kit

How does it help?

It's easy to treat nerves in the privacy of your own home, but you can take your plant compound with you everywhere with a small, discreet travel CBD kit. Sometimes feeling stressed about not having your stress relief can be the worst stress of all! Not anymore.

How to:

1. Sit down with a pen and paper in front of you. What are your CBD needs? Do you have a wrist that gets sore from typing at your desk? A topical can cure that. Anxious workplace? A tincture can treat that. Write down your thoughts.

2. Get a small bag, such as a makeup or toiletry bag. Remember, CBD with THC levels below .03 percent is legal everywhere, so you can take it wherever you want. Pack your CBD essentials into your on-the-go bag. CBD can be pricey, so it's okay if this is the same CBD you use at home.

3. Place it in your purse, backpack, or briefcase. You will never be stuck without your favorite cannabinoid again.

Make Cupcakes

How does it help?

Baking helps you enter a productive meditative state. Amplify this mindfulness activity by creating a shareable CBD treat with this easy cupcake recipe.

You will need:

1 milliliter CBD tincture, 1 box your favorite cake mix, 1 package sugar-free instant pudding mix, 4 eggs, 1 stick room-temperature butter, 1 cup water, cupcake liners, 12-cup muffin tin, your favorite icing, 1 (1,600-milligram) bottle coconut oil–based CBD

How to:

1. Drop CBD tincture under your tongue, then preheat your oven to 350°F.
2. In a large bowl, combine the cake mix, instant pudding mix, eggs, butter, and water together using a spoon or electric mixer.
3. Place cupcake liners in muffin tin. Fill cups with batter and place in the oven. Bake for 15 minutes or until golden brown, then remove from the oven and set aside to cool. Repeat with remaining batter until you have 24–30 cupcakes.
4. Pour your icing into a clean bowl. Stir in coconut oil–based CBD. Then decorate cooled cupcakes with your CBD icing and enjoy.

Stay Hydrated

How does it help?

You may not notice, but staying hydrated is crucial to your mental and physical well-being. Drinking water helps deliver oxygen throughout the body. It also lubricates the joints, reduces headaches, regulates body temperature, helps your digestive system run, and keeps your skin looking great—which are also all benefits of CBD! Practice self-care by making sure you drink 8 (8-ounce) glasses (remember the 8×8 rule) of water per day.

How to:

1. Without breaking the bank, buy a nice water bottle that you are happy to drink out of. Keep it full and with you at all times, whether you're at work or home.

2. Every time you fill your bottle add a squirt of CBD tincture to your water to increase the benefits of this self-care ritual.

3. Drink up and notice how your body functions at its best when hydrated. Once you take care of basic needs such as water, the rest of life becomes easier.

Go on a Walking Meditation

How does it help?

Pair CBD with a walking meditation to step away from worries with less physical discomfort. CBD both eases aches and pains that may arise during a walk and helps you relax into a meditative state. You'll find it easier to be fully present as the CBD reduces intrusive thoughts.

How to:

1. Select a location. It can be your sidewalk, a track at a local high school, a beach, or a nature trail. When you apply mindfulness, anything can become a meditation, including walking. You also get the benefits of exercise.

2. Take your CBD then begin your walk. Use your surroundings to help you stay in the moment. Notice leaves on trees and the sounds of laughter. If an outside thought arises, notice it like a falling snowflake, then watch it melt away.

3. Appreciate your feet for all the work that they do. Experience your heel lifting, and your toes pushing you forward. Calmly breathe in and out. Take a second to appreciate the self-care time that you were able to give yourself with this walking meditation.

Take an Ice Bath

How does it help?

Ice baths help your body recover faster after a hard work-out. They help reduce inflammation (just like CBD!) and flush out metabolic debris you don't need so you can get back in the game. Nervous about the cold? Ease nerves with CBD and speed up healing even more by applying a topical afterward.

How to:

1. Go about your usual workout or gym routine, then consume some CBD when you get home. Opt for a tincture if possible, because the onset time is ideal to create an ice bath.
2. Make your ice bath. You will need 1 (10-pound) bag of ice. Athletes use two, but start small. Pour it into a bathtub filled with cold water. Soak for 10 minutes. You can do it! It's supposed to hurt. No pain, no gain.
3. Once you're out and warmed up, apply CBD topical to sore muscles to further reduce inflammation.

Eat Anti-Inflammatory Foods

How does it help?

Inflammation leads to joint and muscle pain in addition to a plethora of health issues, such as arthritis and sinus infections. Prioritize your health and get ahead of inflammation by combining the anti-inflammatory aspects of CBD with anti-inflammatory foods such as salmon, broccoli, and ginger.

How to:

1. Take some time to figure out what anti-inflammatory foods you'd like to add to your diet. Anti-inflammatory foods include berries, salmon and other fatty fish, garlic, spinach, ginger, broccoli, avocados, and olive oil.

2. Consider how you can increase the anti-inflammatory properties of these foods by adding CBD to your meals. For example, add CBD-infused olive oil to a spinach salad or drizzle some on salmon with avocado. Get creative.

3. Slowly, with the aid of a nutritionist if needed, add these anti-inflammatory foods to your diet and see how you feel.

Sink Into Savasana

How does it help?

Savasana, or Corpse Pose, is the pose of total relaxation. Once you enter such a state, it's a deeply healing form of self-care. Sink into deep relaxation by consuming CBD before trying this yoga pose.

How to:

1. Consume a CBD tincture, then roll out your yoga mat.
2. Sit upright on the mat with your feet flat on the floor and your knees bent. Slowly lean back onto your forearms. Inhale as you extend your right leg and then your left, pushing through your heels. Keep your legs loosely lined up with your hips. Let your feet turn out.
3. Slowly, vertebra by vertebra, unroll your spine until your head and back are gently resting on the mat. Let your arms extend outward by your side. Close your eyes.
4. Notice the earthy taste of the CBD under your tongue. Stay in Savasana for at least 10 minutes. Concentrate on your inhales and exhales, and surrender.
5. When you're ready, exit the pose by slowly rolling over to your right side and gently pushing yourself back up to a seated position.

Wake Up Earlier with CBD Coffee

How does it help?

CBD can sharpen focus and lower stress. In low doses, CBD can even be activating. This dual-action superpower pairs perfectly with coffee, so wake up earlier to feel alert, calm, and productive! Ease into the new alarm time with a jitter-free cup of joe with CBD, which can also act as a treat to motivate you to get out of bed. Too much caffeine can lead to anxiety, but studies show adults can have up to 4 cups a day without issues.

How to:

1. Set your alarm for 15 minutes earlier than normal. If you rapidly try to switch your wakeup time from 8 a.m. to 5 a.m., there's a good chance you'll just keep sleeping.
2. Once you're awake, brew a cup of CBD-infused coffee. Various brands are available online and in stores, but you can make your own by adding CBD tincture or dissolvable powder to your cup of joe.
3. Sit in sunlight as you sip your morning brew. The UV rays are a cue to your brain that it's morning and time to wake up. Sip in silence. Use the coffee ritual as a morning meditation.

Try a Hot Stone Massage

How does it help?

A hot stone massage is done by placing warm stones on the areas of your body that are known to carry tension, such as along the back muscles. The pressure and warmth of the stones help relieve that tension. Taking CBD before a hot stone massage eases you into the most relaxing spa treatment of your life. It can also naturally relieve stiffness and pain by fighting inflammation, enhancing the massage.

How to:

1. Consume some CBD 2 hours before the appointment, or about 30 minutes before if using a tincture. Feel the CBD relieve the stress from your body and help you relax as your massage begins.
2. Fully sink into the experience of the hot stone massage. Feel the weight and warmth of the heated stones placed on your body. Feel the tension release as the hot stones and CBD work together.
3. When you get home from the massage, give yourself the rest of the night off. Immerse yourself in the relaxation.

Go to the Movies Alone

How does it help?

Going to the movies alone is fun and builds independence, but it can still feel unsettling. CBD can help you get over your initial fear, helping you stay present, focused, and fully engrossed in the film without your nerves getting in the way.

How to:

1. Choose the movie you want to see, then head to the theater.
2. There is some stigma surrounding going to the movies alone, but it's a perfect self-care activity. You get to see the movie you want to see. You get to eat all the snacks you want to eat. You get some alone time. However, it can feel stressful to go alone. When you start to feel anxious, consume some CBD to calm your nerves.
3. When the movie ends, congratulate yourself and feel proud. You did exactly what you wanted to do, and that is self-care.

Draw a Homemade Card

How does it help?

Crafting helps your memory and recall skills, and it can even fight against dementia. Get personal by drawing a card for a loved one's next birthday or big holiday. The love and pride from doing something special is a gift to yourself as well. CBD will help you feel creative and let your artist side shine.

How to:

1. Gather your supplies. Break out the scissors, glitter, glue stick, and construction paper. Put newspaper or a garbage bag down to protect the surface that you are working on.
2. Take some CBD and feel your creative side take over.
3. Write a sincere message to the recipient, then have some fun. This card is for someone else, but that doesn't mean that you can't benefit from spreading the love. Express yourself while catering to the audience the card is intended for.
4. Let the card dry, and when it's time, give it to the person you made it for. Enjoy their appreciation of your handmade card.

Do a Body Scan for Physical Self-Care

How does it help?

It's easy to disassociate, or get so stuck in your head or worries that you feel separated from your body. Check in with yourself by conducting a body scan for physical self-care as a dose of CBD tincture dissolves under your tongue. Once you feel relaxed and are fully aware of inhabiting your body—rather than mentally or emotionally floating out into space—you can identify and then treat any pain points that may reveal themselves to you.

How to:

1. Lie down on a flat surface with a pillow under your head. Squeeze a dose of CBD tincture under your tongue. Close your eyes and cycle through a few rounds of deep breaths.
2. Start with your head. Feel the tincture dissolving. How does your jaw feel? Is it clenched? Do you have a headache? Move to your neck. Is it stiff?
3. Continue mentally moving down your body, checking in to identify any physical issues, until you get to your toes.
4. Once you're finished, slowly sit up. Take out a CBD topical and apply it to the parts of your body that hurt.

Make and Use a Massage Candle

How does it help?

Making a CBD massage candle is a mindful self-care activity that activates your senses in order to bring you fully into the present moment. The candle itself is enhanced with the pain-relieving and anti-inflammatory benefits of CBD, and the act of carefully following directions utilizes your ability to focus, which is also amplified by CBD.

You will need:

Candle wick, 4-ounce glass jar, grater, 3 tablespoons natural beeswax or soy wax, 3 tablespoons cocoa butter, 1.6 ounces shea butter, 3 tablespoons sweet almond oil, 1,000 milligrams CBD oil, ⅛ teaspoon (about 12 drops) lavender essential oil (or other scented oil of your choosing)

How to:

1. Put the wick into the jar. Then grate the wax, cocoa butter, and shea butter into small flakes.
2. Make a double boiler by filling a small pot ¼ full of water and bringing it to a boil. Reduce the heat to a simmer and place a heatproof bowl snugly into the pot without touching the water.

3. Add the wax, cocoa butter, shea butter, and sweet almond oil to the bowl. Stir gently for 10 minutes until the mixture is melted, then remove from the heat and gently mix in CBD and lavender oil.

4. Carefully, holding the wick if needed, pour the mixture into your jar and let harden at room temperature for 30 minutes. You can also use 2 chopsticks set across the top of the jar to hold the wick in place.

5. Let the candle cool until it is no longer warm to the touch. Trim the wick as needed.

6. To use, light the candle to set the mood. As it burns, the candle will melt into massage oil that burns at a lower temperature than standard candles. Gently drizzle some over your partner's back or into your hands, and give a massage as you normally would.

Go on a Solo Adventure

How does it help?

Traveling alone, even if it's just a day hike at a nearby park, reminds you of how independent and powerful you are. Of course, solo trips can be intimidating, so use CBD to settle into the experience. Keep some on hand in case worries or fears arise during your adventure.

How to:

1. On the day of your solo trip, wake up by sitting in the sunlight with a cup of coffee or tea infused with CBD. Meditate on your intentions for the day.

2. Pack your CBD and get going! Whether it's a hike, a massage, or a week in Iceland, use CBD to stay in your body and your current settings. Leave your worries at home. This is your time off. Don't ruin it by worrying the entire time. When such thoughts arise, treat them with CBD.

3. Embrace total freedom. This is your chance to have a trip entirely on your terms. Notice how you build confidence and become more independent while traveling entirely on your own. After your trip is over, make an effort to integrate such self-reliance into your day-to-day life.

Rage Journal

How does it help?

Rage journaling is a way to get all your anger, resentment, jealousy, and pent-up stress out of your mind and onto a piece of paper. Journaling about your anger is beneficial but can be emotionally draining. Consuming CBD before and after your writing exercise can help you slow down, focus, and leave those feelings behind on the page when you're finished with them.

How to:

1. Place a few drops of a CBD tincture under your tongue.
2. Grab a pen and journal. Write down everything and everyone that makes you angry. It doesn't need to make sense. Don't worry about spelling or grammar. The words don't even need to be legible. Write until there is nothing angry left to say.
3. After you finish, sit for 1 minute. Place another drop or two of your CBD tincture under your tongue. Rage journaling can be exhausting, but the soothing effects of CBD will ground you and fill you back up with serenity.
4. Sit in silence for a few minutes as the CBD takes effect. Then put your journal away, or rip up and throw out the entries, if that feels better.

Do a Monday Morning Meditation

How does it help?

Monday mornings are hectic, but with the right mindset they can help set the stage for a productive week. Use the anxiety-busting properties of CBD during this guided meditation to take control of Monday morning so you can start your week with a positive outlook.

How to:

1. Ingest your preferred CBD product. Then sit on a yoga mat or pillow and close your eyes. Begin deep breathing. Imagine the CBD attaching to your body's cannabinoid receptors, and welcome a state of calm.
2. Imagine yourself on a comfortable raft drifting down a beautiful river. Feel the water beneath you as it guides your way.
3. Like the river, this week will bring unexpected twists and turns. Trust that it's leading you in the right direction.
4. You know how to swim. Remember that if the current ever feels too overwhelming, you can simply get off and climb ashore.
5. Open your eyes, take a final deep breath, then head off to begin your day.

Socialize

How does it help?
Socialization improves your self-confidence and mental and emotional health, but feeling anxious can get in the way of social activities. Fortunately, studies have shown that CBD treats social anxiety significantly better than a placebo.

How to:
1. Take CBD 2 hours before an event. This gives it enough time to kick in so that when you arrive you are not anxious.
2. Put on your favorite outfit. Wear something that makes you feel confident and powerful. Once you get into your groove and are talking to people, you will notice that socialization boosts confidence as well.
3. Keep CBD with you. Add a few squirts to your beverage to discreetly chill out. Then go have fun. As conversation begins to flow, you will relax. You might even have a good time.
4. Remember that you can leave whenever you need to. Even a little bit of socializing can go a long way for your mental and physical well-being.

Leave an Unhealthy Relationship

How does it help?

Letting go of an unhealthy relationship with a partner, friend, or toxic family member helps you practice self-care by letting go of the past and moving forward to all the joy that awaits. Use hemp rope (available online) and a calming, comforting, stress-relieving CBD tincture to symbolically separate yourself from someone in your life.

How to:

1. Consume CBD, then cut about a yard of hemp rope. Sit on the floor, holding one end of the rope. Place the other end across from you on top of an object that reminds you of your relationship.
2. Allow yourself to feel all the hard feelings. Inhale deeply, then take a pair of scissors and cut the cord in half. Exhale as the rope snips in two.
3. Discard the 2 pieces of rope. Make a concerted effort to move on.

Breathe Away the Day

How does it help?

Stress leads to short and shallow breaths. After a long day, release pent-up tension by trying this deep-breathing self-care exercise coupled with CBD. Settle into relaxation so you can turn off your stress and enjoy the rest of your evening.

How to:

1. Lie on the ground with your head on a pillow. Take a moment to check in with yourself mentally. Are worries flooding your head? Let's get them out.
2. Place a few drops of CBD tincture under your tongue and imagine your worries melting away. You don't need them anymore.
3. Close your eyes. Place one hand on your belly and the other on your chest. Notice any tightness stemming from mental stress.
4. Breathe in through your nose. Let your belly fill with air. Feel your belly button extend upward toward the sky.
5. Slowly exhale out of your mouth. As you do, let your belly drop. Feel it deflate. Blow out the worries. You don't need them. Visualize the ropes of stress coming undone.
6. Continue for 10 minutes. Enjoy the rest of your day from a place of calm.

Make a Budget

How does it help?

The weight of money stress can feel suffocating. Get ahead of financial worry as a form of self-care by building a daily CBD regimen and creating a budget. CBD helps release stress and increases focus, which can help you breathe easier and see your financial planning through clearer eyes.

How to:

1. Consume CBD to sharpen your focus and lower your body's stress reaction.

2. Make a budget. First, use bank statements or an online program to calculate your expenses. Add up your expenses for a year and divide the total by 12 to learn your monthly expenses. Add a 10 percent buffer for emergencies.

3. Now do the same for your income. Subtract your expenses from your income. You should have enough left to put away savings monthly. If not, look for expenses that you can cut.

4. To make paying off debt or building savings easier, set up recurring payments or instant transfers.

5. Make an effort to stick to your budget each month. If you go off track, try to bounce back as soon as possible.

Set an End-of-Day Affirmation

How does it help?

The events of the day can wear on you. Recover mentally and physically by using CBD and setting an end-of-day affirmation. Affirmations are positive statements that fight off negative thought patterns, self-doubt, and stress by reinforcing positive thinking. Stress increases inflammation, but CBD reduces inflammation and lowers your body's stress response.

How to:

1. When you get home at the end of a long day, take CBD. As the calming effects take hold, remind yourself that it's okay to relax. Relaxation keeps you from losing your mind, and it boosts productivity in the long run.
2. Choose your affirmation. It can be personal and specific, or something as broad as "I am powerful. I am loved. What I do is meaningful."
3. Sit in a meditative position, taking a cycle of deep breaths. Begin repeating your affirmation in your head. Continue to repeat your affirmation mentally as you move about your nightly rituals.
4. Use CBD as a sleep aid to ensure a good night's rest.

Search for Your Dream Job

How does it help?

Staying in the wrong job can lead to stress and tension, so practice self-care by searching for your dream job, something that connects to your passions and could transform your life. CBD can help calm down your brain through its interaction with your body's endocannabinoid system, providing a healthy boost of courage to help you job search outside the box.

How to:

1. Take CBD for confidence, then perform an online search. Save job openings that are relevant to your interests, goals, or personal passions. Since you are just looking, feel free to peek at jobs that you may be underqualified for or that are in an entirely different industry from your current career.

2. Update your résumé and apply for a few of those dream positions. Because you are following your passions, be fully honest in your application, and have fun with it.

3. Don't be shy about going on interviews. Even if you don't plan on taking a new job, you can get a glimpse into how industries you've always been curious about operate.

4. If you are offered a new job, congratulations! If not, perhaps you will find a fun side hustle.

Learn about Your Family Tree

How does it help?
CBD users often report that the cannabinoid encourages an open mind by quieting distracting anxious thoughts. Use this creative thinking to actively learn about your family tree. Understanding where you came from may help you better understand yourself, a powerful act of self-care.

How to:
1. Collect anything you can that's related to your family or ancestors. This means photo albums, jewelry, and clothing.
2. Connect with your living family members. What do they know about your ancestry? Do they have stories or additional photos, mementoes, or personal records to share?
3. Consider taking a DNA genetic test. This can show you exactly who your ancestors were and where they came from. You can even find and connect with living relatives you may not be aware of. You can share what you learn with your living family.
4. Visit the grave sites of deceased relatives.
5. Consume some CBD and take time to reflect on what you've learned.

Learn from Your Mistakes

How does it help?

Everyone makes mistakes, but doing so may make you feel awful about yourself. Use CBD to self-soothe, then try this journaling self-care exercise to learn from your mistakes rather than sit and stew and dwell on them.

How to:

1. Place a dose of CBD tincture under your tongue. Let the soothing tincture calm your nerves and any negative thoughts so you can learn from your mistakes.
2. Write down what you did in your journal, such as "I snapped at my coworker again."
3. Now write down why it happened, such as "I haven't been getting enough sleep."
4. Now write down how you're going to learn from your mistake. For example, "I am going to prioritize self-care to be my best self. I am going to focus on my work, which requires me to be friendly and amicable toward my coworkers."
5. Take action and let it go. You are mature enough not to melt down after making a mistake, but to collect yourself, learn, and move forward.

Make and Use a CBD Body Scrub

How does it help?

Make a CBD sugar scrub to exfoliate away worries and dead skin. Making the sugar scrub is an act of mindful self-care, and the use of CBD helps activate your senses of smell, touch, and sight, which anchors you in the now. Making such a lovely self-care item yourself offers a boost in confidence and a feeling of accomplishment.

You will need:

2 (500-milligram) vials coconut oil–based CBD (plus additional for a personal dose), ½ cup coconut oil, 1 cup raw sugar, 10 drops essential oil of your choice such as eucalyptus (uplifting) or lavender (relaxing), Mason jar

How to:

1. Consume a personal dose of CBD prior to the activity. Begin creating your scrub with the intention of being fully present for each step.
2. Melt coconut oil into liquid by heating in the microwave at 15-second intervals until ready or stirring on low heat for 2 minutes in a small saucepan. Once the oil is melted, remove from heat and mix in the sugar.
3. Once the mixture is cool, add coconut oil–based CBD. Then add your essential oil of choice.

continued on next page

4. Add body scrub to a Mason jar, then take a nice warm shower. After the steam opens up your pores, exfoliate away dead skin cells with your homemade CBD body scrub. Store in an airtight container away from sunlight for up to 1 month.

Embrace Your Power

How does it help?

Confidence helps you stand up for what you deserve, feel good about yourself, and reduce negative thinking. Follow this CBD-boosted meditation to visualize yourself in your full power, and let the phytocannabinoid soothe away any self-doubts that stand in the way of the confidence you deserve.

How to:

1. Put on comfortable clothing. Take CBD to get rid of any anxious thoughts.
2. Close your eyes and imagine yourself at the base of a lavishly beautiful staircase. Walk up the stairs.
3. Open the door to a massive room. What is it filled with? There could be rows and rows of books, closets, treasure chests—whatever you desire.
4. The words *I am powerful* fill you. You walk over to a full-length mirror adorned with a gold frame. Look at yourself. Revel in how powerful you look.
5. Spend as much time as you want in this room, and know that you can return whenever you want. When you're ready, walk back down the stairs. Then open your eyes and revel in the confidence that this self-care activity brings out.

Let Love In

How does it help?

It can be hard to let love in. You may often push it away without even realizing that you're doing it. In this exercise you'll open your heart chakra—your spiritual center for love and compassion—with CBD and a mantra. With this self-care ritual you can release the fear that you aren't good enough.

How to:

1. Pull out your yoga mat or pillow, turn on some ambient music, and take some CBD to help quiet any unpleasant or intrusive thoughts.
2. Close your eyes and think about how you may reject love. Maybe you don't even realize that you push it away or how you shut down others. When something nice comes your way, it's hard to trust it, but you must let love in. Think about how you deserve that love in your life.
3. Repeat the mantra "I am worthy of love" over and over. Then imagine a bright-diamond, sparkling light filling your heart. You are worthy of love.

Take Care of Someone Else

How does it help?

Helping others can lower your blood pressure, relieve chronic pain, and give you a sense of happiness and purpose. CBD can help relieve pain and reduce the stress that comes with taking care of someone. It's hard to be the caregiver for someone suffering, and CBD can help take care of you, so you can help take care of them.

How to:

1. Tell your person that you want to take an hour and care for them. Ask how you can help. Practice active listening.
2. Check in with yourself. Taking care of someone is a high-stress, emotional, and labor-intensive job. Take some CBD tincture to keep your stress at bay so you can focus on your loved one without hurting your emotional well-being.
3. Gather supplies based on their needs. Then listen to them. Chat with them over tea. Do their laundry. Cook a meal so that they don't have to. Show them how much they mean to you by showering them with attention.
4. Continue to consume CBD as difficult emotions arise so that you can be your best self.

Explore Lucid Dreaming

How does it help?

Experts say that lucid dreaming—dreams where you can control the outcome—can lead to greater self-confidence and self-realization. Mix CBD with mugwort to stimulate lucid dreaming. Mugwort aids in lucid dreaming and makes dreams more vibrant and colorful, and the CBD fights insomnia and will help ensure you stay asleep long enough to dream.

How to:

1. Keep a dream journal. Jot down your dreams each morning as soon as you wake up. The more you connect with your dreams, the easier it is to lucid dream.
2. Start "reality testing" throughout the day. This includes looking in the mirror, looking at clocks, or pinching yourself to remind yourself that you're awake and not dreaming. When you begin to lucid dream, you can use these same tests to tell that you *are* in a dream—and take control of it.
3. Brew mugwort and drink it as a tea before bed. Take CBD before bed as well.
4. The more you lucid dream, the easier it becomes. Once you control your dreams, you can fight off nightmares and become more in touch with your subconscious, a powerful act of self-care.

Try a Silent Meditation

How does it help?

While most meditations are silent, Vipassana (which means "to see things the way they are") is a silent meditation technique in which you don't speak or make facial expressions or gestures. It helps you see things as they are, which provides clarity, and it reduces confusion, thereby releasing stress. But it's hard to sit still. Use calming CBD to help you focus and sink into the now.

How to:

1. Set a timer for 30 minutes, then drop a dose of CBD tincture under your tongue.

2. Sit in silence for 30 minutes as the CBD kicks in. Let something that's bothering you sit in your mind's eye and observe the issue without judgment. Over the course of your meditation, notice a sense of honest clarity arising.

3. When the meditation is complete, practice self-care by incorporating the acceptance and lessons learned into your day-to-day life.

Release Resentment

How does it help?

Releasing resentment—anger due to being treated poorly—is self-care because it allows you to tackle the emotion and move onward. This requires massive courage, which CBD can help with by lowering your brain's stress response.

How to:

1. Consume CBD, then sit down and journal about your resentment. Be specific, angry, and as long-winded as you like. Get it out.

2. Resentment can be defined as "victim anger." However, as Carrie Fisher said, "Resentment is like drinking poison and waiting for the other person to die." Take some CBD to calm down and identify where your power lies. You can speak up for yourself. You can curate community, love, money, and experience. Meditate on your power. Reclaim it.

3. Using CBD for courage, take action. Speak out. Stand up for yourself. Disconnect yourself from any toxic relationships or people.

4. Make a decision to let go and move forward. This is not letting the other party win. It's about you moving forward stronger than ever.

Practice Aftercare

How does it help?

Aftercare is the simple act of taking care of your romantic partner's emotional needs after intimacy. It helps you and your partner bond. In this self-care ritual, CBD lowers your inhibitions and allows you to facilitate open communication and gentleness.

How to:

1. After an intimate night with your romantic partner, indulge in some CBD. Let the cannabinoid relax you and open your heart to freely share emotions.
2. Check in with your partner. Did they enjoy the evening? Is there anything new they want to try next time?
3. As the CBD lowers your inhibitions and helps shed hang-ups, share your own wants, needs, and desires. The afterglow of intimacy is also a safe space to express your love. Be vulnerable. Tell your partner how much you love them. Notice that when you give love, the act is often reciprocated.
4. Enjoy a deep night's sleep snuggled in your partner's arms. (Remember that CBD is a sleep aid.) Wake up ready to take on the world.

Balance Your Chakras

How does it help?
Chakras are concentrated energy centers in the body associated with various regions, emotions, and modes of healing. Practice self-care by tapping in to this healing mindset through the use of CBD, which reduces negative thoughts and feelings, such as anxiety.

How to:
1. Consume CBD and sit in a chair with your feet firmly planted on the floor. Concentrate on the base of your spine. This is your root chakra. It's associated with survival and safety. Imagine the color red filling this region.
2. Move up to your sacral chakra, located on your lower abdomen. It's associated with sensuality and creativity. Visualize the color orange filling this region.
3. Focus on your solar plexus chakra. This is the chakra of empowerment. Visualize the color yellow filling this area with sunshine.
4. Move up to your heart chakra. It's associated with love and compassion. Visualize the color green, of growth, swelling in your heart.
5. Next is your throat chakra. It's the area of confidence and truth. Imagine the color blue filling your throat with powerful serenity.

6. Focus on your third eye chakra, between your eyes. This is the source of intuition. Imagine it filling with bright indigo purple.

7. Finally, move on to your crown chakra, on the top of your head. This area connects you with the divine. Image yourself wearing a crown of diamonds.

8. See yourself as one. When you're ready, open your eyes and feel like the divine creature that you are.

Try a Bedtime Meditation

How does it help?
When you get a good night's sleep you lower your chances of getting sick, you're able to think more clearly, and you reduce stress and improve your mood. Both meditation and CBD help you fall asleep and stay asleep, so practice this CBD-enhanced bedtime meditation ritual to ensure a good night's rest.

How to:
1. Take out your CBD tincture and place some under your tongue. Feel the earthy goodness absorb into your body and help you enter a state of calm.
2. Sit on the floor, on a yoga mat or pillow, near your bed. Turn off heavy overhead lights and light candles to create a serene environment.
3. Close your eyes and practice a few rounds of regular breathing. When you start feeling relaxed, inhale deeply, then exhale. When you inhale, visualize a glittery, healing silver aura wrapping around each cell in your body and protecting it from harm. When you exhale, visualize any nasty, brownish-green worries blowing out, out, and away.
4. Repeat for 10 rounds (or more if desired), then snuggle into your soft bed, put your head on the pillow, and let your CBD tincture help you sail off to dreamland.

Sit In on a New Church Service

How does it help?

Going to a church service for a religion outside your own can help you expand your mind and become more compassionate. Compassion helps you better understand others, boosts your own self-esteem, and even lowers blood pressure. If stepping outside your typical routine makes you nervous, CBD can help you create a caring, open, and calm mindset to make you feel more comfortable.

How to:

1. Select the service you wish to attend. Is there a religion that interests you? Learn what all the fuss is about by sitting in on a service. Do you have a friend who is of a different religion from you? Learn about their culture. Ask to go together, or make it a solo adventure.

2. Research what to expect, what attire is appropriate, how long the service will last, and other pertinent details.

3. An hour to 2 hours before the service, have some CBD. It will help you relax, allowing you to observe with a calm heart and open mind.

4. Church services are often uplifting experiences. This time you get to experience inspiration from a new source, which can set a positive tone for your whole week.

Unfollow Negative People on Social Media

How does it help?

What you see on social media affects your thoughts and can insert negativity into your life where it doesn't belong. There is no need to follow negative people who fill your timeline and brain with gloomy content, so hit that unfollow button. CBD makes unfollowing (which can be scary!) easier with its calming properties and can help you self-soothe to deal with any lingering negativity.

How to:

1. Take CBD. Defriending and unfollowing people, even those who bum you out, can feel complicated or hard, but it's always for the best. Your life is stressful enough. You don't need to see content that upsets you.
2. Once the CBD kicks in, start unfollowing. Use the block button if someone is harassing you or if you don't want them to see your content.
3. Follow new friends and accounts that make you happy, so when you sign on to social media, it's welcoming rather than stressful.

Get to Know Someone Different from You

How does it help?
Is there someone different from you who you'd like to get to know better? Use CBD to relax and open your mind. Grow your heart and social circle by getting to know someone who scares you.

How to:
1. Decide who you want to get to know. CBD is for making your life more joyful. Pick someone who intrigues you and who you'd like to have as an acquaintance.
2. Have some CBD to calm your nerves. The next time you see them, or have contact with them through email or social media, invite them out for coffee or drinks.
3. Before you meet up, have some CBD. You want to be chill and not nervous. Relax, knowing that they are probably a little shy too.
4. Have some fun. Listen to them. This person is different from you—but that's a good thing. Learn from them. Let them learn from you. Life is more fun when it's filled with diversity.

Have a "Yes" Day

How does it help?
Give yourself an entire day of saying yes. If you never indulge and only deny, the objects of your desire can haunt you and feel like bigger things than they actually are. Adding some CBD to this self-care exercise will help you fight off any guilt you experience from doing things like eating chocolate chip pancakes for dinner or staying out past your bedtime.

How to:
1. Set some ground rules. Perhaps spending over a certain amount or staying up past a certain hour is off-limits. Other than that, for 1 day, you are going to say yes to everything you want.
2. Start the day by ingesting CBD, then make a list of things that you want to do but usually say no to. For example, maybe you always say no to eating a sugary breakfast, wearing a blue wig, or accepting a first date.
3. Commence your day of saying yes! Of course, only say yes to things you want. The point of the celebration is to indulge. If any pesky guilt pops up, use CBD to swat it away.

Try a CBD Sleep Spray

How does it help?

In this exercise, you'll take your self-care ritual into your own hands by making a sleep spray. CBD helps you fall asleep by interacting with the endocannabinoid system and maintaining homeostasis, your body's ability to maintain a state of internal balance and well-being regardless of changes and outside factors. Chamomile is a mild sedative, and studies show lemon balm also treats insomnia. By combining these three safe and natural sleep aids into a sleep spray, you can practice self-care by ensuring yourself a deep slumber.

You will need:

1 (5,000-milligram) bottle CBD tincture, 1 (30-milliliter) bottle chamomile extract, 1 (30-milliliter) bottle lemon balm tincture, 1 (1-ounce) spray bottle, filtered water to fill (make sure to buy edible tinctures rather than essential oils, which are not safe for consumption)

How to:

1. Add equal parts CBD tincture, chamomile extract, and lemon balm tincture to a mixing bowl. Try for 5 milliliters each, but if you can't eyeball it exactly, that's okay. Lightly whisk until thoroughly combined.

continued on next page

2. Use a funnel to pour your CBD sleep spray into a 1-ounce spray bottle. Fill the rest of the bottle up with filtered water. Shake to combine. Spray 3 squirts under your tongue before bedtime to enjoy a great night's rest.

Take a Bath

How does it help?

Baths are a luxurious way to cleanse your body while also easing muscle pain, fighting inflammation, clearing out your sinuses, and reducing stress. Adding CBD oil to the running water during this self-care ritual provides calming anti-inflammatory benefits to your entire body.

How to:

1. After a long day, fill up your bathtub. Adjust the temperature exactly to your liking.
2. Add a few splashes of CBD oil to the warm running water. To make it fancy, add a CBD bath bomb (see "Make and Use a CBD Bath Bomb").
3. Dim the lights. Light candles. Add some bubble bath. Then close your eyes and relax. This time is for you to just sit and relax, nothing more. Soak in CBD and enjoy the self-care until the water cools.

Use a Face Mask

How does it help?
Face masks are fun and relaxing, and they can minimize pores, balance out environmental damage to your skin, and stimulate collagen production. They're also a great source of both mental and physical self-care, especially when combined with the use of CBD oil. This plant-based product can reduce your skin's oil production and treat acne and dry skin thanks to its antibiotic and anti-inflammatory properties.

How to:
1. After washing your face in a hot shower to open up your pores, squeeze a dollop of your favorite face mask into your hands.
2. Add 2–3 drops of CBD oil to the mask.
3. Gently apply the CBD-enhanced face mask according to the package instructions. While it dries, stay away from your cell phone and practice deep breathing to sink into relaxation.
4. Once your face mask has dried, usually about 10 minutes, wash it off using gentle, circular motions.
5. Apply your night cream or moisturizer. Rest well, knowing that you're giving your skin glamorous and modern self-care in the comfort of your own home.

Snuggle with Someone You Love

How does it help?
Cuddling produces oxytocin, the "cuddle hormone," which encourages social bonding and helps you feel happy and emotionally connected to someone you love. CBD enhances this physical self-care exercise by opening you up to your partner's touch and helping you get rid of worries that may prevent you from being vulnerable.

How to:
1. When you're unwinding, make room for alone time with your partner. It's easy to let chores and television push up right against bedtime, so factor in snuggles beforehand.
2. Make sure you're in comfortable clothing on the couch or in bed. Consume some CBD with your partner. Think of a reason you appreciate them. It's so easy for the pettiness of life to trump loving tenderness.
3. Notice how your mind begins to relax. It's okay to let it go and lean against your partner. Have them wrap their arms around you. Stroke their hair. Be affectionate; show them how much they mean to you. Keep it light and don't overthink it.
4. Carry the CBD calm and feeling of love with you as you drift off to sleep in each other's arms.

Relax Post-Workout

How does it help?
It's normal to be a little sore after a tough workout. Muscle recovery takes 24–48 hours, so it's important to rest after exercise. Rub CBD salve into sore muscles to reduce swelling, inflammation, and pain so you can get back out there.

How to:
1. Stretch after your workout. Gently move through a series of recovery postures that address the parts of your body that got a workout.
2. As you stretch, keep a CBD topical by your side. Eliminate outside distractions so that you can be fully present in your body. Notice aches and pains. Gently massage healing CBD topical into these sore areas.
3. Drink plenty of fluids and rest. If you need help reminding your body and mind that it's okay to do so, consume additional CBD to lower your body's stress response.
4. Get a good night's rest. Tomorrow you can return to your active routine.

Get Professional Photos Taken

How does it help?

Feeling like a model for a day offers a major confidence boost—not to mention the resulting photos afterward. Don't worry about nerves. Take CBD before the photo shoot (and keep some on set) for model behavior. The cannabinoid helps make you less inhibited and more likely to loosen up, have some fun, and look your best.

How to:

1. Book a session with a local photographer. Hire a professional hair and makeup artist if your budget allows.
2. Pick out your favorite outfits of all time. Bring multiple looks.
3. Take CBD at least 1 hour before the photo session so you're cool and collected.
4. When you arrive at the studio, ask the photographer to put on your favorite music to help you get into the groove. Then have fun! Give the camera everything you've got. What is there to lose?
5. Take more CBD as needed!

Try a Wrist Massage

How does it help?

In today's busy world, you may find that you're typing on a computer or scrolling on your phone all day, which can lead to common injuries such as tendinitis, or inflammation of the wrist tendon. Thankfully, CBD is a powerful anti-inflammatory, and in addition to treating the cause of the pain, using this natural pain reliever as part of a wrist massage can help you get rid of the pain itself. This CBD massage also helps you practice self-care by helping you remember how important it is to relax, rest, and let your body heal.

How to:

1. Grab your CBD topical. Gently massage it into the sore area, rubbing in gentle circles.
2. As you wait for the topical to sink in, pause and rest your busy hands.
3. Repeat 2–3 times throughout the day as needed. Practice self-care by listening to your body to determine when you need to rest. Keep your CBD topical nearby and use it to prevent future aches and pains.

Learn about Your Sun Sign

How does it help?

Astrology is a great way to have fun and reflect on your personality and relationship and thought patterns. See how the stars align for you by learning and reading about your sun sign. CBD suppresses the fight-or-flight response—which new experiences, however safe, may cause—and allows you to sink into the now.

How to:

1. Take CBD to relax. It's okay if you're not sure about astrology. Just have some fun, the ultimate form of self-care!

2. Your sun sign is determined by the position of the sun at the time of your birth. If you don't know yours, just search online. All you need to know is your birthday.

3. Ask yourself what traits of your sign resonate with you? Which do not? Use this astrological information as a tool for self-reflection and consider your thoughts, patterns, and relationships.

4. If you're having fun reading about your sun sign, learn about your moon sign or the sun signs of other people in your life.

Unwind in Candlelight

How does it help?

Turn off electronics and turn on candlelight to create calming ambience. CBD's stress-busting powers can help you ease into a relaxing analog atmosphere by affecting the areas of the brain that regulate stress. CBD also interacts with your brain's serotonin production, encouraging calm and boosting mood.

How to:

1. Make room for a candlelit night of relaxation on your calendar. When you arrange things ahead of time, you're less likely to ditch your plans.
2. Stock up on candles. While simple white pillar candles will do, feel free to pick unique colors and scents that make you happy.
3. Prepare food, drink, and CBD before getting started. Once your self-care spread is ready, scatter the candles around your home. Light them. Turn off all the light bulbs. Put away your phone to avoid ruining the mood.
4. Take your CBD, eat food, and drink wine (if you like) in the candlelight. Notice how calm and at home you feel. You're tapping in to your primal nature. Enjoy.
5. Before you go to bed, remember to blow out every single candle.

Plant a Garden

How does it help?

Studies show that gardening decreases your dementia risk, combats loneliness, and counts as aerobic exercise. It's also an amazing self-care exercise, as it can relieve your stress by helping you connect with nature. CBD can enhance this practice by working to boost your mood and using its anti-inflammatory benefits to keep your hands and fingers nimble as you plant and pull out weeds.

How to:

1. What do you want to grow? This is your garden. Do you want flowers to decorate your home? Herbs to add to cooking? Or all the above? Self-care means doing what you want.
2. Consume some CBD orally to invite in that signature focused calm.
3. Get dirty. Plant seeds, pull weeds, and water. Use your arms to reach and pull and bring new life into the earth.
4. When you are finished for the day, take a long, hot shower, then gently massage your topical CBD into your wrists, hands, and fingers.
5. Continue to integrate CBD into your gardening self-care practice and watch your plants sprout and grow.

Heal a Hangover

How does it help?

Hangovers happen, and making sure to take the time to properly care for yourself when you're feeling unwell is the epitome of self-care. Fortunately, CBD can help you. It eases the pain of a headache and relieves nausea, while also reducing hangover-related anxiety.

How to:

1. One of the reasons hangovers are so painful is dehydration. Fill up a giant glass of water and start drinking. Grab some electrolyte-rich drinks, such as sports drinks or coconut water, to ramp up the recovery.
2. Add CBD tincture directly to your drinks, or place it under your tongue in between beverages.
3. If you can, take the day to rest. Let yourself off the hook and catch up on movies or a TV show. Keep drinking fluids, and wake up the next day restored.

Draw a Self-Portrait

How does it help?

Drawing a self-portrait is a creative way to express yourself, connect with your identity, and discover new personal traits. It can give you a sense of control, boosting your self-esteem while stimulating your creativity and intuition. And if you're feeling insecure, CBD can help you work through that insecurity and boost your confidence level.

How to:

1. Take a few deep breaths and some CBD. You are safe in this moment to be your creative self.
2. Take out your notebook, a mirror, a pencil, and an eraser. Begin drawing. Don't worry about the right place to start or draw—just start.
3. Drawing yourself can feel strange, so if you are unhappy with how you look, change it! A self-portrait does not have to be a mirror image of yourself. It's all about how you feel.
4. Check out your work. Self-portraits can offer valuable insight into your self-esteem and how you view yourself. If you like, reflect on what you learned by taking notes in a journal or on a piece of paper to help process your feelings.

Care for Your Hair

How does it help?

Not only does caring for your scalp and hair make you feel more comfortable, it makes you feel fabulous. When you look good you feel good! CBD can help enhance this self-care exercise because it is full of fatty acids that nourish your hair, and the cannabinoid's anti-inflammatory properties treat dandruff, eczema, and itchy scalps.

How to:

1. Squeeze your shampoo in your hand, then mix 2–3 drops CBD oil directly into the shampoo.
2. Wash your hair. Be sure to spend time gently massaging your scalp to enhance blood flow and stimulate new hair growth while strengthening your current locks. (See "Give Yourself a Scalp Massage.")
3. Rinse out the shampoo, then condition as usual. While the conditioner sits, enjoy the steam from the hot water. Steam clears out your sinuses to prevent colds, clears up your skin, and even burns calories. It can also help you feel great and relaxed as you practice self-care.
4. When you're done, rinse out your conditioner, then continue your day or night as usual, knowing that you've taken some time to care for yourself.

Get Organized

How does it help?

Research shows that a clean house leads to a happy mood. And when you clean up, you feel productive and effective, which provides an immediate mood boost. Fortunately, CBD can both help you focus and ease any emotional stress that comes from letting go of the past. It will enhance this self-care ritual by keeping you stress free as you create a clean and organized environment.

How to:

1. Begin by having some CBD to help you focus. Try a tincture, which will kick in quickly, after about 15–45 minutes.
2. Make a list of what needs to be tackled. Break it down by room or project.
3. Keep going until you've reached your limit or have finished your list. Afterward, apply a CBD topical to stay ahead of any aches from your hard work.
4. Revel in your beautiful, clean home. Remember, cleaning provides a feeling of confidence and accomplishment, so take the time to enjoy it!

Try Legs Up the Wall Pose

How does it help?

CBD-enhanced yoga is a perfect way to practice self-care because it helps you relax, clear your mind, and focus solely on yourself and your body. The inverted nature of this pose also helps the body circulate blood and further promote relaxation. Additionally, this pose works to regulate digestion, which is also a benefit of CBD.

How to:

1. Place your yoga mat on the floor with the short end up against a wall. Sit down, relax, and take a CBD tincture. This will take about 15–45 minutes to kick in, allowing you to gently enter a calm yoga mindset.

2. Lie down with your legs up on the wall, then shimmy your hips closer to the wall until they're as close as they can get. Your body should make an L shape.

3. Let your arms fall by your sides, then practice a few rounds of deep breaths. Breathe in, breathe out, breathe in, breathe out. Let your pelvic floor relax. As your spine is decompressed, feel the tension in your lower back float away.

4. Do you feel calm from your CBD? Let your worries fade away along with the tension as you honor your body.

Make and Take CBD Gummies

How does it help?

CBD's neuroprotective properties help reduce damage to the brain and nervous system while encouraging the growth and development of new neurons. This means that CBD could prevent the progression of neurological disorders, reduce cell damage, and promote healing. Use these beneficial CBD gummies as a snack, as needed for pain relief, or as a daily supplement. All these usages work to help you take a moment to care for your body.

You will need:

½ cup chopped fresh peaches, 1 teaspoon honey, ½ cup water, 8 teaspoons unflavored gelatin, 250 milligrams CBD oil tincture, silicone candy mold

How to:

1. Use an immersion blender to thoroughly combine the peaches and honey in a mixing bowl. Then set aside.
2. Pour water into a saucepan. Sprinkle the gelatin on top. Let sit for 2 minutes, then stir and place over medium-low heat. Continue to stir until the mixture combines, which should only take a few minutes.
3. Pour gelatin mixture on top of peach mixture and stir well. Stir in CBD.

continued on next page

4. Gently pour mixture into candy mold. Refrigerate for 30 minutes or until cool and firm.
5. Pop out the gummies and enjoy. They will stay fresh in the refrigerator for 2–3 weeks.

Build a Fort

How does it help?

Whether you're at work or at home, you probably have to act like a grown-up all day long. Playful activities, such as building a fort, can help you relax, get silly, and have some fun. Fortunately, adding stress-busting CBD to this playtime will help you tap in to your childlike curiosity and shed any hang-ups about adulthood.

How to:

1. Consume some CBD and gather your fort-making supplies. You can use chairs, blankets, sheets, couch pillows, or whatever else you have around your home. Don't worry about looking silly. This is all about having fun and creating a temporary space just for you!

2. Try arranging the chairs in front of your couch. Remove the couch cushions to turn them into walls. Hang the blankets and sheets over the couch and chairs to create the fort roof. Place other pillows, blankets, books, and toys inside the fort.

3. Use the fort for fun and snuggles with family members or pets, or as alone time to cozy up with a good book. Either way is self-care!

Pick Your Battles

How does it help?
Annoying things happen every day, but choosing your battles preserves your energy for when you truly need to metaphorically pick up arms, which makes this a mental self-care exercise. CBD calms anger to help you know when to fight for yourself and when to let it go.

How to:
1. If you find yourself getting angry, take some CBD to ground yourself. Then look at the problem objectively. Be ready to admit when you're being petty, and walk away from the issue if you are.
2. If the issue at hand is one worth having a conversation over, consider the timing. Your friend or partner is going to be more amicable during the day in person rather than late at night over text. Then bring up the issue from a constructive, assertive, and calm mindset. Actively listen to your partner. Admit when you're wrong. If the conversation becomes stressful, have some CBD.
3. Use all efforts to end on a constructive note. Make a plan to use going forward to prevent this issue from arising again.

Limit Your Caffeine

How does it help?

Too much caffeine can lead to anxiety, agitation, and difficulty sleeping, none of which help with self-care! Focus on being the calmest, most healthy you that you can be by using CBD to help limit your caffeine intake. CBD eases caffeine withdrawal symptoms, helps you sleep better, improves focus, and can even act as a non-habit-forming caffeine substitute. Add a CBD tincture to beverages such as green tea, which contains 12–20 milligrams of caffeine as opposed to coffee's 40–120 milligrams.

How to:

1. Set self-care goals. How much caffeine do you currently drink, and what is your goal? It's better to cut back slowly than go cold turkey. For instance, for 1 week, switch out your morning coffee for some CBD green tea.

2. When you need a caffeine pick-me-up, brew a cup of green tea, then add 1 milliliter of CBD tincture and enjoy! Think about how great you feel as you sip your self-care.

3. Make note of how you feel after 1 week. Further reduce your caffeine intake, aided by CBD, if you like the results.

Exchange Neck Massages

How does it help?

If you keep a great deal of tension in your neck—a common problem if you work at a computer—nothing will feel more decadent than a neck massage from your partner. Exchange neck massages using CBD oil, which is both pain relieving and anti-inflammatory. It can help you relax and ease pain while helping you connect with your loved one.

How to:

1. Have your partner get into a seated position, either on a chair or cross-legged on the floor, so you have full access to their neck and back.
2. Put a squirt of CBD oil in between your hands and rub them together to warm the oil.
3. Knead your thumbs into your partner's sore muscles. Communicate to learn what stroke style and pressure they like.
4. After 15 minutes, swap places with your partner. Relax and let your partner rub out your tension and neck pain. Allow yourself to enjoy the intimacy of making each other feel good, and relish in the time that you're spending taking care of you.

Use an Immunity Booster

How does it help?

While we need more research to understand how and why, CBD is believed to fight carcinogens and boost immunity. This may be due to its anti-inflammatory properties. This recipe mixes CBD with echinacea, vitamin C, and other immunity boosters that will help you stay sharp and healthy. Keeping yourself healthy is an important way to practice self-care, so plan a preemptive strike with CBD and care for yourself by getting ahead of colds before they get you down.

You will need:

8 ounces orange juice, 1,000 milligrams CBD tincture, 1,000 milligrams echinacea tincture, 1 tablespoon elderberry syrup, 1–2 ice cubes, seltzer water to fill

How to:

1. Pour your favorite orange juice into a tall glass. It should be about ⅔ full.
2. Add CBD tincture, echinacea tincture, and elderberry syrup.
3. Add in an ice cube or two and fill the glass to the top with seltzer. Stir vigorously. Drink up and know that you're prioritizing your self-care practice by taking care of your health!

Enjoy Essential Oil Aromatherapy

How does it help?

Aromatherapy can aid in digestion, promote relaxation, improve sleep, and manage pain—powerful self-care benefits! CBD shares these benefits and can enhance your aromatherapy practice by strengthening the self-care elements of your essential oils.

How to:

1. Place some full-spectrum CBD oil in your hand. What does it smell like? Different forms of CBD have different terpenes, or organic aromatic compounds that are responsible for a strain's unique smell. The smell of these terpenes will help you decide which type of essential oils to pair with your particular type of CBD, and what the benefits of your aromatherapeutic self-care will be.

2. If your CBD smells musky and earthy, you're likely inhaling myrcene, a terpene known for its analgesic and sedative effects. Mix with lavender essential oil and place under your nose to inhale calm.

3. If your CBD smells like citrus, that's the terpene limonene. It fights anxiety and balances mood. Mix with lemon essential oil and place under your nose for a boost of energy unadulterated by anxiety.

4. If your CBD has a cooling smell, that's cineole, also known as eucalyptol. It's found in eucalyptus, and research suggests it can improve cognitive function.

5. Continue to mix and match CBD oils and essential oils until you create custom blends ideal for your needs. To use, place 1 drop of oil under your nose to breathe in directly. You can also add 1,000 milligrams of oil in a spray water bottle to spritz your pillow, bedroom, or even your office.

Care for Your Lips

How does it help?

Your lips can become uncomfortably dry, especially in the winter, if you've been exposed to UV rays or if you're not drinking enough water. Dry lips can lead to flaky skin and inflammation, and they're a constant reminder of how you're not taking the time to take care of yourself. This quick and easy CBD self-care exercise helps you treat dry lips and remind yourself how important you are.

How to:

1. Purchase CBD lip balm. Look for a product made with full-spectrum CBD, which is packed with the most nutrients possible.
2. Rub the tip of a cotton swab on the CBD lip balm. Gently massage the cotton swab over your lips to remove flaky skin and create a smooth base to moisturize.
3. Then apply the CBD lip balm directly to your lips. Wait 10 minutes or so before eating or drinking so your lips can soak in the nourishing CBD.

Savor Dessert

How does it help?
While eating in moderation is good advice, it's important to treat yourself and splurge sometimes. Not only does having dessert taste good, but it can boost your mood, just like CBD! Use CBD to stimulate your appetite and help you focus on the moment so you can savor every bite of your favorite dessert.

How to:
1. After you finish eating dinner, relax for 30 minutes or so to let your food digest, then place a few drops of CBD tincture under your tongue, or add some to your post-meal coffee or tea.
2. Be still while the CBD begins stimulating your appetite and enhancing your senses. Rather than turn on the TV or look at your phone, try doing nothing.
3. When you're not so full from dinner, bring out your favorite dessert. Whether it's a cookie, chocolate, or pie, agree to have 1 piece without any guilt.
4. Enjoy the treat bite by bite. Let CBD help you focus all your attention on how delicious it tastes. You deserve it.

Go to Bed Early

How does it help?

Going to bed early can help you get enough rest and function at your full capacity the next morning. Turning in rather than staying up can be tough, especially if you're breaking a routine, but prioritizing your well-being is an important aspect of self-care. Fortunately, the sedative and calming properties of CBD can ease the transition.

How to:

1. Set a bedtime for yourself. Pick an earlier time that is not too different from your current bedtime.
2. Brew yourself a cup of caffeine-free tea. Then add 1 milliliter CBD tincture to the brewed tea. You can also add the tincture to hot water with lemon or just take it by itself.
3. Find something low-key and calming to do as the tincture kicks in. Sit somewhere cozy, read a book, or listen to some calming music.
4. Take a moment to stretch before bedtime. Apply CBD topical to any sore aches or pains.
5. Tuck yourself in bed at your new bedtime and let CBD carry you off to a lovely slumber.

Give Yourself a Foot Massage

How does it help?
Your feet have a demanding job—they carry you everywhere! Thankfully, giving yourself a foot massage enhanced with an anti-inflammatory CBD topical can relieve foot pain and help you manage discomfort. Plus, it just feels absolutely fantastic, a wonderful benefit of physical self-care.

How to:
1. Take out your favorite CBD topical or add a few drops of CBD oil to your favorite moisturizer.
2. Remove your shoes and your socks. Be sure to keep a pair of comfy new socks nearby.
3. Rub the topical in your hands to warm it up, then start massaging the arches of your feet with your thumbs.
4. Move on to your toes. One by one, massage each toe. Concentrate on the joints, which can get stiff and are easily inflamed.
5. Move to your heels, which can dry up and crack easily. Slather on the CBD, then put on your fresh pair of comfy socks. This way your feet can absorb all the pain-relieving moisturizer.

Curl Up in a Blanket

How does it help?

It can be hard to let go of your day and simply relax. But taking the time to curl up in a nice blanket helps you feel warm and protected. You can enhance these feelings by enjoying a dose of de-stressing CBD before you snuggle up.

How to:

1. Invest in a quality blanket. Do you want a big, fluffy white comforter, like what you'd find at a hotel? Or maybe a weighted blanket, which can be a great choice for relaxation? Weighted blankets ease anxiety, insomnia, and stress.

2. Once you have your blanket, grab your CBD and a good book if you like. Consume some CBD to help yourself de-stress from the day and enter relaxation mode.

3. Snuggle up. Wrap yourself up in your blanket. Allow yourself to soak in the comfort. Your job is simple but important—enjoy some rest and relaxation. Read, meditate, or simply drift off to sleep.

Relieve a Headache

How does it help?

From stress headaches to migraines, throbbing temples are all too common. They can get in the way of work, your exercise routine, or your ability to be present with a loved one—and they hurt! Practice self-care by prioritizing your physical health, and treat your headache naturally with pain-relieving CBD.

How to:

1. When your mind is busy, it's easy to ignore head pain because you're not connected to your body. Take the time to ground yourself with a few deep breaths.
2. Sit down. Put on something soft. Set up the environment to make yourself as comfortable as possible.
3. Take some CBD as soon as possible. Ingest it orally via tincture or capsule. You can also rub some topical on your temples, or wherever it hurts.

Clear Up a Breakout

How does it help?

Acne breakouts are often caused by stress, because when cortisol (the stress hormone) increases, so does oil production. And it's tough to feel your best when you think your skin looks its worst. Fortunately, CBD's anti-inflammatory properties can help treat acne and breakouts by lowering your cortisol levels and clearing up your skin.

How to:

1. Wash your face, then apply CBD oil or a CBD-based product to the affected area.
2. Follow up your skin treatment by applying a moisturizer. If it's during the day, use one with an SPF. If it's at night, opt for a night cream.
3. Ingest CBD orally to lower your stress levels, and be sure to carve out time for additional types of self-care.

Stimulate Your Appetite

How does it help?

Sometimes when you're stressed, not feeling great, or really busy, it can be easy to forget to eat. But when you're not fueling your body, you're not going to feel your best, and your focus, energy levels, and metabolism will all be negatively affected. Practice physical and mental self-care by using CBD to stimulate your appetite, sharpen your focus, and function at your maximum capacity.

How to:

1. Place a few drops of CBD tincture under your tongue. This should encourage your appetite while also curating calm. Once the tincture has kicked in (about 15–45 minutes), choose what you want to eat.
2. If you're coming off a period of time when you weren't eating, beverages such as smoothies or protein shakes are great ways to get your nutrition in. Add a CBD tincture to elevate your beverage.
3. As you get your appetite back, continue to practice self-care, including getting enough calories. Remember to make yourself a priority in your own life.

Calm Your Stomach

How does it help?

Whether you're suffering from gas, cramps, constipation, or something else, stomach issues can be embarrassing and can distract you from everything else you have going on. Thankfully, CBD treats the disruptive effects of an upset stomach, leaving you free to go about and enjoy your day from a place of comfort and confidence.

How to:

1. First identify the cause of your upset stomach. Is it something you ate? Stress and anxiety? Do you have a stomach bug? Go see a doctor if needed.
2. To settle your stomach, place CBD tincture under your tongue, or add 1 milliliter to seltzer or another sparkling beverage.
3. Let CBD help you relax. Snuggle up somewhere you can be alone, and give yourself a break. Engage in a relaxing activity like watching TV or reading a book.
4. Once you're feeling better, treat yourself to a healthy snack or a cup of tea.
5. Going forward, keep track of what upsets your stomach, and how CBD can help.

Enjoy a Mindful Cup of Tea

How does it help?

You can turn any self-care ritual into a meditation by practicing mindfulness, the psychological process of becoming fully present in the present moment. Mindfulness keeps you in the "now" so you can experience your joyous life fully rather than becoming bogged down in anxious thoughts about the past or future. Like CBD, chamomile tea is famous for its relaxation properties, so add a dose of CBD tincture to a cup of calming chamomile to unwind and practice self-care.

How to:

1. Gather chamomile tea, honey, and your CBD tincture. Minimize outside distractions. Focus entirely on the present.
2. Boil water. They say a watched pot never boils, but mindfulness asks you to be in the now and trust that everything will work out. Take this time to focus on smells, the sound of boiling water, and other happenings in your home, and relax into the now.
3. Prepare your cup of tea. Place a chamomile tea bag in your cup and a dollop of honey if you please. Inhale the earthy scent of the tea bag and the sweetness of the honey.

continued on next page

4. Pour hot water into your cup. Let the tea steep for about 5 minutes. Sit somewhere comfortable and practice several cycles of deep breaths to help keep you in the present.

5. Squirt 1 dropper, or 1,000 milligrams, of CBD tincture into your tea, then stir. Hear the click of your spoon as the CBD mixes with the herbal tea and honey. Slowly sip your cup of relaxation and practice self-care by remaining fully in the moment. Stay away from electronics as you savor each taste of the relaxing sweet herbal goodness. This time is for you and you alone.

Go to a Concert

How does it help?

In addition to the joy of seeing a band you love perform right in front of you, attending a concert helps you practice mental self-care by ensuring a good time with your friends. CBD calms any intrusive, anxious thoughts so you can dance ecstatically, fully present in the moment, while enjoying the soul-nurturing sounds of your favorite band.

How to:

1. Check out the shows in your area, invite your friends, and buy tickets.
2. There can be nerve-racking aspects of seeing live music. Crowds can be sweaty and pushy. Sometimes you have to wait in line. If you feel nervous about heading out, consume CBD prior to the concert, and turn your focus to having fun rather than worrying about what may happen. Bring some additional CBD with you in case you need some during the show.
3. Have fun! Dance, socialize, sing along with your favorite songs. Enjoy your self-care!
4. After the show, unwind with a CBD bath to soak off the sweat and engulf your sore muscles in the healing power of the cannabinoid.

Travel

How does it help?

Travel can reinvigorate your lust for life, expand your understanding of the human experience through new cultures, and grant a deepened appreciation of your life back home, but the planning, actual travel time, and being away can be nerve-racking. Fortunately, CBD can calm your nerves and decrease any physical issues so you can enjoy this self-care experience. CBD can also fight nausea, which is common on airplane flights, car rides, and even train rides.

How to:

1. Plan and book your trip. Choose something fun that will expand your mind and work as spiritual self-care. Take some CBD at home before you leave.
2. If you're flying, try edible CBD to calm your nerves. Edibles can take up to 2 hours to kick in, but will last for up to 8 hours, which will get you through the security line and your flight.
3. If you're driving, depending on how CBD affects you, you may want to hold off on consuming CBD until you reach your destination. Then relieve the stress of a road trip by unwinding with a CBD tincture.

Host a CBD Dinner Party

How does it help?

Friendships boost your health and happiness, and can make difficult life events easier. Practice self-care by laughing, eating, and bonding with your loved ones over a nutritious meal that's infused with relaxing CBD, so everyone can unwind and de-stress together.

How to:

1. It's easy to let friendships sit on the back burner. However, when life gets hard, it's friends who see you through to the other side. Create a guest list and send out invites to your CBD-infused dinner party.

2. Plan and execute the meal. Don't be afraid to ask for help. These are your friends, after all.

3. Before the dinner party, take some CBD to help you stay present and relax.

4. After everyone arrives and you bring out the food, introduce the CBD. Keep different tinctures around, such as an olive oil–based CBD tincture to add to savory dishes or dip bread in, a coconut oil–based tincture for sweeter creations, or an alcohol-based tincture to transform a cocktail. Let your friends play with CBD as they dine and enjoy the company.

Smash Something

How does it help?

Anger is not a negative emotion. It's just an emotion. If you shove it down or ignore it, it will only fester and rear its ugly head at undesirable times. Pent-up anger can lead to stress, high blood pressure, and irritable moods. Get rid of those feelings by safely smashing your worries. Then use calming CBD to help you self-soothe afterward.

How to:

1. Select a towel and something to break. A glass works well, or you can play it safe and opt for a hard plastic cup.
2. Roll the item up in the towel, then grab a hammer.
3. Use your hammer to break the glass through the towel. Go hard. Let out all your anger. Scream as much as you want.
4. Safely clean up the remains of your at-home anger workshop, and think about how much better you feel. Consume some CBD to invite in calm after the storm.

Dive Into Diaphragmatic Breathing

How does it help?

Diaphragmatic breathing is deep breathing done by contracting the diaphragm. CBD will help you relax and focus before you begin sinking into diaphragmatic breathing. The breathing and herbal relaxation will help you center yourself, become aware of your power, and fight anxiety with spiritual confidence.

How to:

1. Squeeze a dose of CBD tincture under your tongue. Then, in a comfortable seated position, place one hand on your chest and one hand below your rib cage. Notice any energy blockages, or areas that feel like dull gray clouds restricting your energetic flow.
2. Breathe in slowly through your nostrils. Let your stomach expand out against your hand. Imagine that you are inhaling a silver white light of power and serenity.
3. Tighten your abdominal muscles, letting them move inward while you exhale. Keep the hand on your upper chest as still as possible. Imagine that you are blowing out any gray, black, or sickly green-colored tension bogging you down.
4. Repeat for 10 rounds. Allow calm to wash over you. Keep it with you throughout the rest of your day or evening.

Organize Your CBD

How does it help?

Organization aids in time management, increases productivity, and reduces stress. Keep your CBD accessible and well organized for a beautiful display and easy access. You can also use this opportunity to express yourself creatively by creating a setup perfectly tailored to your needs.

How to:

1. Consume CBD via your preferred method and decide if you want to keep your CBD in plain sight or out of view. If you want to keep it tucked away, keep your topical with your beauty products, your capsules with your vitamins, and your tinctures in your medicine cabinet.

2. If you want your CBD all in the same place, obtain a container for safekeeping. This could be a basket, a cabinet just for your CBD, or a storage bin slid under the bed. Trust your instincts!

3. Go ahead and organize your CBD. Admire it and feel good about taking the time to organize something that's just for you.

Combat Dryness

How does it help?

Dryness can leave your skin feeling like a desert. Fortunately, taking the time to care for your skin with CBD can be an amazing self-care ritual. CBD regulates oil production and blood flow, leaving your skin feeling great, nourished, and glowing.

How to:

1. Take a warm shower to relax, cleanse, and open up your pores. The steam helps eliminate toxins, clear sinuses, and enhance circulation.

2. Even though you're out of the shower, get ready to get messy. Stay naked if you have the privacy.

3. Squirt your favorite moisturizer into a bowl, then add CBD oil (at your desired strength). Mix the two together until fully combined, then transfer the mixture to a Mason jar.

4. Rub the CBD lotion into your feet, legs, hands, shoulders, and any other area where you experience dry skin.

5. Sit in casual meditation while your body absorbs the CBD moisturizer. Let your mind focus solely on your skin. Then, after a few minutes, put on comfy clothing and spend the rest of the evening loving your glowing skin.

Have a Picnic

How does it help?

Picnics are a fun way to get out of the house and into the sun, and spending quality time with loved ones helps you live your best life as friends and family offer positive advice and feedback. Make this social self-care even more enjoyable by using CBD to help everyone shake off everyday stress and more fully enjoy the time together.

How to:

1. Find an afternoon when you are free and the weather is nice and sunny. Invite friends and family whose company you enjoy. Planning any group activity can be stressful, so take CBD as needed.
2. Go to the grocery store and stock up on delicious and healthy snacks for the picnic. Find a balance between fruit such as grapes, savory snacks like cheese and crackers, and sweet snacks like cookies.
3. If you are the CBD connoisseur of your group, bring along some tinctures, CBD beverages, or capsules to try. Start a discussion on how CBD helps you. And, of course, don't forget to have fun with your friends!

Create an Aphrodisiac Tincture

How does it help?

Reconnect with your partner and enhance intimacy with a CBD aphrodisiac tincture. Making the tincture is a mindful self-care activity that can help you feel extra loved and cared for both as you make it and as you enjoy it. CBD can enhance emotional connection and keep you focused on the present moment. It can also help you feel better in your body by increasing blood flow and lowering pain.

You will need:

1 (16-ounce) glass canning jar, dried rose petals, dried damiana leaves, 1,000 milligrams CBD tincture, about 12 ounces grain alcohol such as Everclear to fill, cheesecloth or fine-mesh strainer, smaller clean and empty tincture bottles

How to:

1. Fill your jar ¾ full with dried rose petals, damiana leaves, and CBD tincture. Rose petals act as heart openers, and damiana is a stimulant that enhances excitement.
2. Pour grain alcohol over the herbal mixture all the way to the top, then screw the lid on tight. Store in a cool, dark place for 1 month.

continued on next page

3. Take out your tincture. Strain through cheesecloth or a fine-mesh strainer into a small bowl.

4. Divide up among small tincture bottles or rebottle in another glass jar. Place 1 drop of tincture under your partner's tongue and have them do the same to you. Revel in the shared intimacy of a homemade loving aphrodisiac, and appreciate how good this intimacy makes you feel about yourself.

Let Go of a Grudge

How does it help?
Grudges keep you angry and stuck in the past. Prioritize yourself by releasing resentment and moving forward with a light spirit. Letting go of grudges isn't easy. It requires great emotional strength and intelligence. Knocking away stress with CBD helps you be the bigger person and do the right thing.

How to:
1. Get comfortable, with some CBD to subdue hard emotions, and get to the root of your grudge. Who are you mad at—and why? It's easy to let go of resentments after properly identifying them.
2. Communicate. You can have more CBD if needed. Talk to the person you're mad at. It's the only way to get rid of the grudge. If you don't free it through communication, it will dig deep down inside you and fester.
3. Feel your feeling. Sadness or anger are not bad emotions. They are just emotions. The only way out is through.
4. Decide to let it go. You can forgive, but you don't have to forget. This is about getting on with your life.

Go Shopping

How does it help?

Shopping is excellent cardio in addition to being a whole lot of fun, but feet get sore and crowds are stressful. CBD helps you manage your time and shop more efficiently by lowering stress levels and increasing focus, helping you hit up all the stores you want to visit.

How to:

1. Malls and stores can be overwhelming, so write down what you want ahead of time. Then take some CBD and get ahead of sore feet by applying CBD topical to your soles and toes.

2. Shop! Let CBD calm any anxious thoughts that may arise. You're shopping because it feels good—and you already know what you're looking for and what you have to spend, so there's nothing to feel nervous about.

3. When you're done, collect your loot and head home. Shopping can be a workout, so practice self-care by taking a warm bath with a CBD bath bomb or oil. Soak so your entire body benefits from the pain-relieving, relaxing, and anti-inflammatory benefits of CBD.

Make a Power Playlist

How does it help?
Music is a healthy and natural mood booster—just like CBD—so practice self-care by creating and then playing a playlist of all your favorite uplifting songs. Dancing and singing is encouraged and will further raise your serotonin levels.

How to:
1. Put on your favorite happy song. As you dance around your home, consume some CBD to gently lower your inhibitions and get you into a happy and relaxed mood. If your dance moves cause any aches or pains, apply CBD topical to the area.
2. Now open your computer and make a power playlist. Add the song that made you dance. Continue to add songs until you have about an hour of feel-good tunes. If the song lifts your spirits, add it.
3. It might be just a playlist, but these few songs have the power to change your entire mood. When you feel cranky, hurt, sad, or lethargic, take some CBD and turn it on. Use CBD to silence any negative thinking and remind yourself that you're as powerful as your playlist.

Get a Routine Checkup

How does it help?

Sometimes the stress of not going in for a checkup is worse than the stress of going to the doctor. Practice physical self-care by using CBD to shake off any medical fears and then get checked out to make sure you're in tip-top shape.

How to:

1. Have some CBD to calm your nerves, then book an appointment with your primary-care doctor for a routine checkup.
2. It's okay to have some CBD before your visit. It's also okay to talk to your doctor about hemp and CBD. Be open and honest with your doctor about anything and everything that is bothering you.
3. After you get home from the doctor, treat yourself to a CBD lollipop or edible. Then relax, knowing that your doctor's visit is out of the way. You don't have to do it again for an entire year.

Try a New Workout Class

How does it help?

A change in workout activates different muscle groups and can help prevent injuries that occur from using the same muscles over and over. Don't fret about soreness from using your body in new ways—that's what CBD is for. CBD is pain relieving, yet doesn't numb you. Some evidence suggests that CBD can speed up muscle recovery, and it can alleviate any anxiety you may have about trying a new workout class, which can be scary!

How to:

1. Workout classes allow you to feel like a child again. However, starting a new fitness class may leave you feeling like a new kid on the first day of school. Consume some CBD to relax and allow yourself to fully immerse yourself in the class.
2. Have fun, focus on the music, and appreciate all that your body is capable of doing.
3. New forms of exercise make you use different muscles, which can leave you sore. Apply a CBD topical to any sore areas such as the lower back, knees, and shoulders after the class.

Binge-Watch TV

How does it help?
It's hard to allow yourself to do nothing. In today's society, everyone is programmed to constantly be on the go. Fortunately, a night in watching TV helps you take the time to rest and reboot. Use CBD to help your body relax and enjoy the show.

How to:
1. First, get comfortable, then take a CBD capsule or two. It will help heal aches and pains. The stress-busting properties of the cannabinoid also let you forget work and worries.
2. Select a TV show to binge. It's time to start a new guilty pleasure.
3. While you're at it, order a food delivery or break out the snacks. CBD invigorates the appetite, so get ready to eat.
4. Relax and enjoy the show, knowing that doing nothing is exactly the self-care that you need in the moment.

Volunteer at an Animal Shelter

How does it help?
Working directly with animals lifts your spirits, and you'll feel good about yourself for doing something good for others. You might feel sad about how many animals need a family, but CBD can help lower your stress levels and help you be your best self around the animals.

How to:
1. Perform an online search to find animal shelters in your area. Call and find one that's looking for volunteers.
2. Choose what type of service you wish to provide. You can help socialize the animals by playing with them, drive them to vet appointments, or aid in adoption. You can also foster pets straight from your home.
3. Take some CBD tincture before you begin volunteering to take the edge off, allowing you to relax and enjoy the animals' company and the honor of the work.
4. Continue to take CBD as needed while you are there. Seeing all the animals who need homes may be upsetting. Use CBD to help you stay positive so you can give the animals your best self.

Book a Hotel for the Night

How does it help?

Spice up your normal routine (and consider surprising your partner) by booking a room. Even if you're only a few blocks away from home, a night away will help you relax and leave your everyday worries behind. CBD helps make this possible by quieting intrusive thoughts and helping you stay present.

How to:

1. Pick an occasion. Do you and your partner or friend have a birthday, anniversary, or Valentine's Day coming up? Search for hotel deals in your area to celebrate. But you don't need a reason to enjoy a staycation. Sip some green tea laced with CBD tincture while you browse.

2. Get to the hotel room early. If it's a romantic stay, spread some rose petals on the bed. Bring a CBD tincture to rest on the bedside table.

3. During your staycation, you must both agree to let go of the outside world. Use CBD to open up emotionally, safely lower inhibitions, and calm the mind. Exchange massages with a CBD topical.

Make Your Childhood Dream Come True

How does it help?

Hobbies help fight stress, promote mindfulness, and can connect you with others and help you make new friends. Fulfilling your childhood dream can also boost your confidence and make you feel like a rock star. CBD can help you focus and create an actionable plan and stay motivated in case you feel like giving up.

How to:

1. Take a little bit of CBD, and remember what you wanted to do as a child. Identify your youthful dream career. Now do research into the best way to experience it. If you wanted to be a firefighter, look into becoming a volunteer firefighter. If you wanted to be a ballerina, take adult ballet classes.

2. Make a plan that realistically works with your schedule, and then follow through. If you feel like quitting, call on CBD's motivational benefits. Don't buy a package of 12 painting classes and then show up for only a couple.

3. If you get nervous before your reentry to childhood, calm down with a higher dose of CBD.

Sleep In

How does it help?

While it's nice to get up early, it's also nice to sleep in when you can. Catching up on sleep is associated with better memory, less inflammation (CBD is an anti-inflammatory too!), better heart health, and lower stress. Fortunately, CBD is a known insomnia treatment and can help you luxuriously sleep in on the weekends to recharge.

How to:

1. Stress and racing thoughts may be keeping you awake. Let CBD ease your worries by taking 25–1,500 milligrams before bedtime. If ingesting orally, take 1–2 hours before bedtime. If using a tincture, take it 30 minutes to 1 hour before bed.
2. Turn off your alarm clock. Put your phone on sleep mode. Put fresh sheets on your bed, and consider an eye mask and ear plugs. White noise machines can also help keep you sound asleep.
3. Keep CBD near your bed to take if you wake up in the middle of the night or too early. It will help you fall back asleep.
4. Sleep in and do not feel guilty about it. Revel in this self-care activity and wake up refreshed.

Boost Your Intuition

How does it help?

When you're in touch with your intuition—subconscious thinking that relies on knowledge and previous experience to give you a gut feeling—you can make more effective decisions, avoid poor choices, and live your best life both in love and at work. Not sure how to feel more intuitive? A daily meditation can help. CBD can help you knock out intrusive thoughts and quiet your mind during your meditation so you can be fully present in the moment.

How to:

1. Set aside 10 minutes a day to perform your self-care meditation.
2. Sit on your yoga mat or a pillow. Drop a dose of CBD tincture under your tongue.
3. As the herbal remedy gets to work, filling your mouth with the taste of plant elixir, close your eyes and begin deep breathing. Continue until a sense of calm floods your body and mind.

continued on next page

4. If there is a specific topic you need insight on, tell yourself while meditating that the answer is already inside you. You simply need to trust your intuition. Eventually an answer will arise. A thought floats to the forefront of your mind, and you realize that you knew the answer all along. You are a powerful being; sometimes you just need to carve out time to reconnect with yourself and your intuition.

5. Continue your daily CBD meditation—set a goal of doing it once a day for 30 days. Notice how your intuition develops.

Face Your Fears

How does it help?

The more you face your fears, whether it's asking for a raise or saving a spider, the braver and more confident you become. CBD can help you feel strong enough to try new things as it lowers your anxiety by binding with your endocannabinoid system, helping you be your best self.

How to:

1. Consume CBD, then think about which fear you want to overcome.
2. Make a pros and cons list. What's the worst thing that could happen? Have you survived worse already? What's the best thing that could happen? If the best-case outcome excites you more than the worst-case scares, then go for it.
3. If needed, take some additional CBD, then do the thing you're afraid of. Agree to a public speaking event. Book a flight and get on the airplane. Enjoy the feeling of empowerment that comes from facing your fears!

Do a Forward Bend

How does it help?
The spine, neck, and back are prime pain centers. Tension builds up in these areas when you type, text, do chores, feel stressed out, and more. Fortunately, you can relieve this tension by doing forward bends, which stretch the hips, hamstrings, calves, thighs, and knees while keeping your spine strong and flexible. Use a pain-relieving CBD topical to help you relax and access this useful pose at home or even at work.

How to:
1. Stand up with your feet together. Bend your knees gently. Slowly begin falling forward vertebra by vertebra. Bend from your hips and not your back. Anytime you feel discomfort, take a break and rub CBD oil onto these spots.
2. Stretch your hands toward the floor, then lift your kneecaps and gently spiral your inner thighs to straighten your legs.
3. Feel your neck elongate as your crown falls toward the ground.
4. When you're ready, slowly roll back up, vertebra by vertebra. Take a moment to feel the stretch affecting your body, and acknowledge how good it feels to take time for yourself.

Read a Book

How does it help?
CBD helps you focus and stay calm and present, allowing you to turn off your worries and to-do lists as you lose yourself in a good book.

How to:
1. Carve out reading time in your schedule. If you don't, you risk putting reading on the back burner and missing out.
2. Pick a book that is unrelated to work, family, or any stressor. Pick one that is purely entertainment. Go for fiction, science fiction, historical fiction, or whatever genre brings you joy. You are reading a book for self-care.
3. Set yourself up with some CBD. Ingest it directly, or add a tincture to a nice cup of tea to sip while you read.
4. Move electronics away from your sacred reading space. No social media or other distractions allowed.
5. Get cozy. Snuggle up on the couch or a comfy chair with a blanket in case you get cold.
6. Start reading! Consume more CBD as desired.

Make a Scrapbook

How does it help?
Scrapbooking is an act that can help you practice mindfulness and express your creativity. As a bonus, it leaves you with the gift of preserved memories. CBD's calming effects can help you unleash your creativity, and CBD can also help sharpen your focus, allowing you to be fully present as you craft.

How to:
1. Pick up a scrapbook, pens, stickers, glue, tape, glitter, or any other crafting supplies that make you happy. Be sure to pick a theme. Do you want to honor a friendship or relationship? Is this a scrapbook of all your travel adventures?
2. Consume CBD and set up your crafting space.
3. Go nuts. Glue. Cut paper. Write in the corners. The point of a scrapbook is to have fun while memorializing your life. Really pay attention to what you're doing in the moment. Enjoy organizing the pages, and remember how the memories you're scrapbooking made you feel. Appreciate the mindful time that this self-care exercise has given you.
4. If your scrapbook honors one relationship, consider giving it to the other person as a thoughtful and personal gift.

Set Boundaries

How does it help?

Good boundaries (the healthy limits you set with other people) make for healthier relationships. Loving relationships can lower blood pressure and stress and boost your immune system. Use CBD to sink into this self-care meditation, which will help you strengthen your personal boundaries.

How to:

1. You can't set boundaries if you don't know what yours are. Consume CBD and sit cross-legged on the floor or on a yoga mat.

2. Close your eyes. Inhale and exhale 10 times. Ask yourself: What feels intrusive? What feels unsafe? Keep a pen and notebook nearby to jot down the thoughts that arise.

3. Close your eyes, breathe deep, and visualize your boundaries like a nice, safe fence that keeps intruders out. Your boundaries keep you and your relationships safe from harm.

4. Once you've realized what your boundaries are, discuss them with the other parties in question. Be ready to enforce them. Those who love you will respect you for it.

Take a Break from the News

How does it help?
Today, thanks to social media, it may seem like you are plugged into the stressful news cycle 24/7. This type of constant stress can damage neurons and even shrink your brain—but the damage is reversible. Fortunately, CBD helps you stay present and off your phone, and can help relieve stress. It even encourages neural regeneration.

How to:
1. Choose a day to take a news break. Turn off your phone notifications, keep the TV off, and honor your commitment.
2. Consume CBD. Allow yourself to forget about what you may be missing and be mindful about what is actually going on in the world around you. If you're stressed about missing a breaking story, CBD helps alleviate such fears. If anything truly important happens, someone will tell you.
3. At the end of the day, reflect on your stress levels and how staying away from the 24/7 news cycle affected your mood.

Keep a Dream Journal

How does it help?

Dream journals can boost overall memory, stop nightmares, and help you sleep more deeply. Certain terpenes in full-spectrum CBD products are associated with higher dream recall, such as terpinolene, which can reduce sleep problems; limonene, which can reduce insomnia; and pinene, which helps you fall asleep faster. Let CBD help you keep a daily dream diary to better understand and track what's going on in your unconscious.

How to:

1. Use CBD as a sleep aid to ensure a good night's rest. When you wake up write down whatever you remember, even if it's just a singular image or a feeling. Give your dream a name. This tool is used by sleep researchers to aid in memory recall.

2. Throughout the day, more details may come back to you. Welcome them and add them to your dream journal.

3. At the end of the day, reflect on the details of the dream you had the night before. Does it contain metaphors for your waking life? How can your dreams offer you helpful insight? Notice how your memory improves and how you have better control over the content of your dreams.

Step Away from an Argument

How does it help?

Avoid getting heated or saying something you regret in an argument by stepping away for a moment. By not immediately reacting, you practice self-care by allowing yourself time to gather your thoughts, calm your nerves with CBD, and then return to the discussion.

How to:

1. If a fight feels like it's escalating or is just generally unproductive, take a minute and step away. Then consume CBD to help calm down. Reflect on what you're angry about. Take some deep breaths.

2. Check in with your body. How do you feel? Your body can help give you clues about your emotions. For instance, a tightness in your chest can indicate hurt. Muscle tension is a reaction to stress. Your body is preparing you to go to battle, so to speak. Take some deep breaths, shake your body out, and remind yourself that everything is okay and there is no real threat.

3. Return to the person you're arguing with. Assertively express your concerns in a calm manner. Speak directly to what you're angry about. Your goal is to come to a peaceful resolution.

Make and Use CBD Bath Salts

How does it help?

Bath salts cleanse the body of impurities and improve circulation, and the addition of CBD adds an anti-inflammatory benefit to the list. It's hard to apply topicals all over the body, but by adding them to the bath, you can coat your entire self in relaxation. Additionally, the act of making your own self-care tools adds a mindfulness practice to this self-care bathing ritual.

You will need:

1 (16-milligram) dropper CBD oil, 2 cups Epsom salts, 10 drops lavender essential oil (or your favorite scent), Mason jar

How to:

1. Take a moment to place a few drops of CBD oil under your tongue to focus and ease into the moment.
2. In a mixing bowl, combine Epsom salts, the dropper of CBD oil, and lavender oil. Stir gently until all the ingredients combine. Inhale the relaxing scent.
3. Transfer bath salts to a Mason jar.
4. Run a warm bath and add 1 cup homemade CBD bath salts. Let your entire body relax in the calming and purifying water. Store your bath salts in an airtight glass container, and they will last for years.

Try Reiki

How does it help?

Reiki is a form of energy healing that relieves pain and tension while restoring energy blocks. Use CBD to relax and keep an open mind, then practice self-care by clearing out your heart chakra, which is located in your chest. The heart chakra is associated with compassion, love, and beauty.

How to:

1. Sit cross-legged on the floor or on a yoga mat. Drop your desired amount of a CBD tincture underneath your tongue.

2. Close your eyes. Place your hands over your heart. How does this area feel? Your heart chakra may contain immense emotional pain from current or past hurt. Does it feel hot to the touch? Do certain colors come to mind? Do you feel repressed emotions rising to the surface?

3. Reiki is a universal healing energy. You are already connected to it, even if parts of you need love and healing. Imagine a silvery pink light. Harness it with your hands and press the loving-kindness into your chakra. Hold your hand against your chest until you feel nurtured and joyous.

Write a Poem

How does it help?

Writing poetry can act as a self-care tool that turns your emotions and pain into art. CBD can help you both access and process your emotions, and it will help you let your guard down and write powerful poetry.

How to:

1. Sit somewhere cozy. Self-soothe with CBD. Most people come to poetry to express their emotions, so acknowledge what you are feeling. What's happening in your body? Is your chest a knot of pain? Or are you so happy that you feel like you're floating?

2. Take out your pen and paper. Begin writing offline to avoid the stress of screens. Don't worry about rhyming. Just start freestyling. This poem is just for you. It can be as weird, dark, or obsessive as you like. The goal is to work through your emotions and turn them into art. If you want to clean up the poem later, do so in an edit session.

3. If you want to share your poem, use some CBD to calm your nerves, then give or read the poem to a trusted friend or loved one.

Cheer Up on a Rainy Day

How does it help?

Rainy days can be gloomy. But since they may make you want to stay inside, rainy days are perfect for self-care rituals such as reading, taking a bath, or playing with pets. CBD can help boost serotonin levels, boosting your mood so you can appreciate rainy days and get the most out of your self-care.

How to:

1. Sit by a window. Consume some CBD as a mindfulness aid. Look outside and count all the things that make you happy, such as the sound of rain hitting the pavement, powerful lightning bolts, and the smell of the rain. There's even a word for it—*petrichor*, "the smell of fresh soil after rainfall."

2. Turn your attention to inside your home. Count what you're thankful for, such as your family, pets, a good book, and cozy blankets to curl up in.

3. Think of rain as a metaphor. Like hard emotions and situations, it comes, and then it passes. It has beauty if you're willing to observe. And when it's over, you get sunshine, happy plants, and even a rainbow.

Do a Body Scan for Spiritual Self-Care

How does it help?
Your spirit is your truest form, so emotional pain can manifest as what feels like a dark cloud in your chest or a throat that feels blocked. Practice self-care by taking time to be fully present in your body and observe where you need to send yourself extra self-love and care. CBD can help you shed any worries or anxiety and will allow you to fully inhabit your body as you scan for spiritual pain.

How to:
1. Consume some CBD using a tincture. Lay out a blanket or yoga mat and gently lie down on your back.
2. Close your eyes. Feel the CBD melting under your tongue. Take a series of deep inhales and exhales.
3. Start at your feet. How do they feel? Wiggle your toes. Continue to breathe. Tell each part of your body that you love it. Thank your feet for carrying you around all day long.
4. Mentally, slowly move up your body. Use visualization skills to notice areas that feel blocked or hurt. For instance, if you are anxious, your chest may feel like a tight black knot. When you feel this, place your hands on the area. Visualize yourself sending healthy, pure light to the area to heal it. You are going to be okay. Let the loving energy heal the spiritual cracks or hurt you feel.

continued on next page

5. Move all the way up to your scalp. When you are finished, take some time to rest. If any areas of your body feel sore, gently rub some CBD topical onto them.

Redecorate

How does it help?
Redecorating your home with colors and objects that make you happy gives you a mood boost that has lasting effects. Research suggests that CBD increases blood flow to the brain, which is associated with creativity—a necessity for redecorating.

How to:
1. Take CBD to boost creativity. Make a mood board, a collage of images that will inspire a space and represent the goal you wish to accomplish.
2. Look into the meaning behind colors. Blue is for tranquility, red for passion, pink for self-love, yellow for joy, orange for creativity, purple for royalty, and green for abundance. Which colors speak to you?
3. Research basic feng shui tips. Declutter and make sure there is good energy and air flowing through your home.
4. Set a budget, then start shopping for supplies. You can go as big as new furniture or as small as adding flowers to a space.
5. Don't get stressed out! Redecorating is an exciting way to change the mood of your home, which affects your mood. Have fun with it!

Give Yourself a Day of Rest

How does it help?

Today everyone is so busy that it's easy to forget to make time for rest, which is why you should practice self-care by scheduling a day for just that—and sticking to it. Researchers say that a day off can lower your stress levels and fight inflammation—just like CBD can! Use your CBD as a sedative to help you unwind.

How to:

1. Cozy up on your couch, take some CBD, and remind yourself that you need downtime.
2. If your life is very active, try to fit some sleep and well-earned laziness into your day of rest. Sleep in. Cook a big, delicious breakfast. You can even get food delivered. Catch up on your favorite TV show or read a book. Take a long, luxurious bath. Do whatever you want! It's your day of rest.
3. Work 1 day of rest per week into your schedule as often as you can. You deserve it!

Cook with CBD

How does it help?

Cooking is an act of mindfulness that will bring you fully into the present moment by utilizing your senses. It is an art and a science that asks you to trust your instincts and follow instructions. CBD not only amplifies your mindfulness and focus but can be added to most savory dishes, leaving you with a delicious and nutritious reward that nurtures your body, mind, and soul.

How to:

1. Select a recipe to follow, then choose your ingredients.
2. Consume CBD before and as you cook. Make cooking an active meditation. As distracting anxious thoughts fade away, focus entirely on the smells and tastes. Take advantage of this opportunity to connect with the senses. Deeply inhale. Focus all your energy on smell. Notice sizzling and other sounds. Taste your food. Let the flavors mingle and marry on your tongue.
3. Enjoy the fruits of your labor (and feel extra relaxed as you enjoy them thanks to CBD!).

Release Your Creative Blocks

How does it help?
Research shows that making art can cause your stress levels to drop, and creativity helps you express yourself. Unfortunately, energetic blocks can stand in the way of your art and self-expression. The good news is that research suggests that movement and creativity are linked—and CBD stimulates creativity. So pair CBD consumption with this walking meditation to restore your creative flow.

How to:
1. Take CBD to relax, then close your eyes and deeply breathe at your own pace. Remind yourself that the idea that will burst your creative block is already inside you. It will appear when it's ready.
2. Find a safe location where you can walk around for 10–15 minutes. Feel free to dance, do jumping jacks, skip, or walk your dog. All that matters is that you get your endorphins going.
3. Let your mind be fully present in the moment. The more you let go, and let CBD and endorphins flood your body, the more readily creative answers will come your way.
4. Get to work on all those wonderful ideas coming your way!

Cancel Plans

How does it help?

You're exhausted. You want to save money. You worked all day and don't want to go out again. Practice self-care by prioritizing your needs and canceling that date or get-together. Use CBD to get rid of any guilt that you feel about canceling, and honestly communicate your needs to your friend or partner.

How to:

1. You need to cancel plans because you're stressed. Don't add to the stress by stressing about canceling! Have some CBD, and as your worries begin to disappear, reach out to your friends.
2. Don't lie about having a dentist appointment or family emergency. Be honest, explain how you're feeling, and ask to reschedule. Feel good about being able to vocalize what you need and making yourself a priority.
3. Make the most of your night in. Eat what you want, watch what you want, and get plenty of rest and relaxation.
4. Honor your rescheduled plans. Canceling for a night of self-care is important, but nurturing and maintaining your relationships should also be a priority.

Make a Floral Arrangement

How does it help?

Making a flower arrangement allows you to express yourself creatively and connect with the natural world while activating your senses. CBD can help you focus on your arrangement by getting rid of distracting thoughts and helping you be totally present.

How to:

1. Consume a CBD tincture, then head to your local florist.
2. At the florist, follow your senses to pick out the right flowers for you. Engulf yourself in the sight, the smell, and even the feel of the flowers. Pick ones that speak to you. Then pick out greenery and baby's breath to fill out the arrangement.
3. Back home, pour water into a vase. Then cut away an inch of the flower stems and any extra leaves that will fall below the water level of the vase.
4. Add the largest flowers first in a circle. Then move on to the next biggest, and when the flowers are done, add the baby's breath and greenery.
5. Place the flowers in your home, and revel in the natural beauty you created. Thank yourself for making your home an angelic space.

Ask for Help

How does it help?

When you are run-down, overwhelmed, or in need of a day off, you may just push through it and keep going, but ignoring your needs won't help you in the long run. Practice self-care by using CBD to open up emotionally and let others know when you're at your limit and need help.

How to:

1. Know when you feel overwhelmed. Be realistic. Be honest. Learn to recognize your limits before you have a panic attack or feel tears coming on.

2. When you feel you've hit your wall, step back and assess the situation. Whether it's physical exhaustion or a shortened fuse, identify indicators that you need some self-care stat. Keep CBD with you. Take it to calm stress and to remind yourself that everything is going to be okay.

3. Self-care is important, but sometimes self-care means leaning on your support system. Reach out to someone you trust, and ask for help. Accept the help without guilt. You can make it up to them when they need your help.

Accept the Things You Cannot Change

How does it help?

There are some things that you cannot change, no matter how hard you try. Practice self-care by letting go of what is out of your control. Acceptance is not defeat but rather the recognition that it's time to choose another, better path. Letting go is hard and stressful, but CBD can soothe your nerves and help usher in acceptance.

How to:

1. Take some CBD and get out a pen and paper. Write down everything that you're upset about. It can be on a small scale, such as something your spouse did. Or it can be grand in scale, such as an environmental disaster.

2. Look at each item and identify what you can change. For example, you could reduce your own environmental impact. Make a plan to put those changes into action.

3. Then identify what you cannot change. For example, you can't control how the rest of the world lives. Focus on what you can control, such as expressing love to your friends and family, how well you do your job, and more.

Strengthen Your Core

How does it help?

A strong core acts as the foundation for your whole body. It can reduce your risk of injury and can help stop some aches and pains. Taking the time to focus on core-strengthening activities will improve your posture, balance, and even brain power. While strengthening your core can be tough work, CBD helps you avoid pain and feel self-confident. Just remind yourself that it feels good to be strong, but you're already beautiful.

How to:

1. Sip some CBD-infused water.
2. Lie on a yoga mat and place your feet flat on the mat, hip-width apart, with your knees bent. Cross your arms over your chest. Contract your abs and inhale through your nose.
3. Exhale, and lift your upper body toward your knees. Keep your head and neck relaxed, and use your abdominal muscles to do this lift.
4. Inhale, and lower yourself back down, vertebra by vertebra. Repeat for 3 sets of 20 crunches.
5. If you're sore afterward, apply a CBD topical.

Stop Racing Thoughts

How does it help?

Don't let stress bleed into the free time that could be used for relaxing. Here you'll couple CBD with a deep breathing exercise to stop racing thoughts—intrusive, repetitive, anxious thoughts that make it hard to focus on anything else. This will lower your anxiety levels and allow you to be mindfully present in the moment, a form of mental self-care.

How to:

1. Take CBD and sit somewhere quiet. Practice the fourfold breathe, which is fabulous for calming anxiety. Breathe in for 4 counts, hold for 4, exhale for 4, and hold for 4. Repeat for several rounds.
2. After a few cycles, practice deep breathing at your own pace. Mentally say the phrase, "I am safe, I trust the process of life." Keep this mantra with you at all times, and when racing thoughts about a touchy subject arise, take control. Replace the intrusive words with the kind mantra. You are safe. Everything will work out the way it should. Return to your breath, and know that you're practicing mental self-care by choosing to remain calm.

Soothe a Short Fuse

How does it help?

A short fuse can be a sign of exhaustion—and a sign that you're not spending enough time practicing self-care. Fortunately, CBD can help you both self-soothe and get a good night's rest so you can wake up and treat others the way you'd want them to treat you.

How to:

1. Check in with yourself. Are you tired? Hungry? Make sure your basic needs are being met. Take some CBD.
2. As you feel the CBD start to take hold, get into bed and get a good night's sleep. Then wake up and eat a healthy breakfast.
3. Take some quiet time to check in with yourself. Are you still snapping? If so, ask yourself when it started. Was there a particular incident? Are you still upset about it? If that's the case, have a calm yet assertive conversation with the other person in question to work things out or make needed changes.
4. Apologize to the people you snapped at. Make amends when needed. Keep CBD around to help you practice self-care when you feel stress build in the future.

Prevent Burnout

How does it help?

Dealing with burnout—feelings of exhaustion, difficulty concentrating, and shortness of temper—when you're already struggling is one thing, but mapping a course to avoid burnout before it begins is true self-care. Burnout makes you less productive in the long run, so form and implement a plan to stay ahead of it with the relaxing effects of CBD.

How to:

1. Take some CBD, then figure out how and when to use CBD on a daily basis.
2. Work exercise into your weekly routine. Make a commitment to yourself to go to the gym, on a walk or run, or to a fitness class a few times a week and stick to it.
3. Rely on your support system. Make time for friends, lovers, and family.
4. Identify your professional goals. Burnout gets worse when you feel like you're mindlessly following orders. If you're working toward a goal that's important to you, it's easier to stay excited and optimistic about work.
5. The next time you feel exhaustion and burnout creeping in, remember that you are one step ahead with your self-care plan.

Make a Pros and Cons List

How does it help?

Making a list of pros and cons about a situation helps you discover your true thoughts and come to the best decision for your life. Studies show that CBD addresses the stress response, helping you calm down and see situations clearly.

How to:

1. Take some CBD to quiet any anxious and distracting thoughts that have come up about the situation at hand.
2. Take out a pen and paper and make 2 columns, one for pros and one for cons.
3. Get the bad news out of the way first. Write down every possible con related to the situation. Then move on to the good. List all the possible pros.
4. Look at the list. Which has more entries? By the end of this exercise, your true desires will be obvious. Act on them. Use CBD for a boost of confidence if needed.

Embrace Your Independence

How does it help?

Independence boosts your confidence, lightens the load on your friends and family, and helps make you financially secure. But it is easy for self-doubt and negative thinking to get in the way of your independence. Fortunately, CBD gets rid of the anxious thoughts that work to prevent you from living your life free as a bird.

How to:

1. Place a dose of CBD tincture under your tongue. As it dissolves, mentally tick off all your best attributes. Are you strong, brave, smart, and committed? Have you survived horrible situations before and come out on top? Remind yourself of everything you like about you. Take a pen and paper and make a long list. Look at it and add to it regularly.
2. Practice making decisions all by yourself. Make a decision entirely on your own and see how it goes.
3. Independence is sexy. Watch how people respond to you differently as you become more independent and embrace the life you live, standing on your own two feet with loved ones by your side.

Accept Criticism

How does it help?

Take the time to better yourself by accepting constructive criticism with an open heart and mind. Research shows that CBD can lower stress and the fight-or-flight response, which can help you stay grounded and consider feedback from a level state of mind.

How to:

1. The next time someone criticizes you, step back for a minute before reacting. Take some CBD to help calm down and focus on the critique.

2. Be brutally honest with yourself. Is this person trying to bring you down? Or do they care about you and are they only trying to help? Look at your internal reaction to the criticism. Can you separate facts from emotion? Scan your emotional reaction to see if you are trying to rationalize your mistake or make excuses. Both are unhelpful. When you view the matter as an impartial witness, is the feedback helpful? Can you benefit from it?

3. Ask the other person about the criticism. Listening to the "why" can take away the sting, and even provide useful feedback so that you do better next time.

Acknowledge Shades of Gray

How does it help?

As easy as it is to believe that things are either good or bad, that's not how people or situations are in real life. Everyone exists in shades of gray. Acknowledging this fact, with the aid of calming and mind-opening CBD, makes life less painful. When you're able accept that sometimes people mess up—or that someone or something is not pure good or pure evil, but real and messy—you'll become more compassionate and forgiving of both yourself and others.

How to:

1. Use CBD to enter a state of mindfulness. Notice how you judge others or situations as "good" or "bad." Some things, such as acts of violence, are undeniably bad. But people, such as your romantic partner or boss, are likely not so easily categorized.

2. Acting judgmental takes up a lot of energy. Wouldn't it be easier if you accepted that everyone contains both good and bad?

3. The next time you find yourself quick to judge someone, have some CBD to welcome in compassion. Think about what upset you. Yes, it is difficult, but is the person in question always a source of negativity? Do they have qualities that bring you joy? Have you ever acted in a similar manner? If you can forgive yourself, can you forgive them?

4. Try to remind yourself of shades of gray on a daily basis. You are not evil for making a mistake, and neither is anyone else. You are just human, and you are perfect in your imperfections.

Identify Triggers

How does it help?

Triggers are certain topics or words that make you uncomfortable or remind you of painful memories. Stay one step ahead of the stress that triggers can cause by taking CBD and identifying what triggers a panicked response for you. This way, you can politely excuse yourself from situations that make you feel uncomfortable.

How to:

1. Sit down with a journal and pen. Consume CBD to self-soothe.
2. Make a table with 3 columns. Label them "Trigger," "Emotion," and "Coping Skill." In the Trigger column, note what words or fears cause an intense emotional reaction—for instance, the name of your partner's ex.
3. In the Emotion column, write down how each trigger makes you feel—for example, "jealous and sad."
4. In the Coping Skill column, note a strategy to manage emotions when that trigger arises. For example, write down "reality check" to remind yourself that your partner is with you and that relationship is in the past.
5. When a trigger arises, practice self-care by utilizing the coping skill you've identified for that particular trigger.

Shower Cry

How does it help?

Researchers believe that shower crying feels good because you are safe and comforted. Practice self-care by letting go of sadness, and the pain and resentment it can cause, in this safe place. Release your fear and stress with CBD. Research shows that CBD can help your brain stimulate the growth of new neurons, which both reduces stress and helps your brain let go of the past.

How to:

1. You had a long day. You're suffering inside. That's hard. Take some CBD tincture. After about 15 minutes, head to the shower.

2. Turn on the shower water as hot as you like. Get in. Let the steam open your sinuses and reduce stress.

3. Let it out. Cry as hard as you can. If it's comfortable, sit down in the shower. Let the warm water run over you as the tears wash down your eyes. Cry until there's nothing left.

4. Use the shower as a safe space as often as you need to. When you repress emotions, they remain trapped inside you. The only way to move past them is to let them out.

Dress Up for Date Night

How does it help?

Dressing up for date night helps you feel confident and can keep the romance alive in your relationship. When you show respect for the event—the romantic night out—your partner will respond appropriately, with admiration and respect. If you feel silly dressing up, CBD can help you get rid of those nerves and help you feel more confident, like the rock star you are.

How to:

1. Take CBD, then make sure all the details of your date night are in order.
2. Be brave while getting ready. Wear an outfit that brings out your confidence. Don't worry about looking vain or silly. Squeeze your date night for all that it's worth.
3. If you have any clothing or jewelry that reminds you of your partner, wear that to increase the bond between the two of you.
4. When you're ready, and it's time to go on the date, practice mindfulness and active listening. Listen to how your partner is doing, share your life updates with them, and open up emotionally. Use CBD to stay fully present and make the most out of each moment.

Write a Love Letter

How does it help?

CBD reduces the fear response and allows you to be bold and put yourself out there. Use that confidence to make someone else's day with a handwritten love letter. Expressing love helps you feel more loved too.

How to:

1. Take CBD. Sit somewhere comfy where you can meditate. As the CBD starts to take effect, think about how much you love this person. If anything they do annoys you, breathe through it.

2. Keep a notebook by your side. As you reflect, jot down notes. How does the person you love inspire you? How has your life changed for the better since they joined it? Do you have anything sexy to say?

3. Sit down to write the love letter. If you don't know where to start, just start writing. Words will come. It doesn't have to be perfect. It just has to be honest.

4. Read the letter back to yourself. Feel the love. Revise and edit if you like, but remember that it's okay to be messy and real.

5. Give the letter to the one you love. Embrace the joy felt all around.

Give Yourself a Full-Body Massage

How does it help?

Your body is a temple. Treat it like one by practicing self-care and massaging it with the pain-relieving and anti-inflammatory properties of CBD.

How to:

1. Sit cross-legged on a yoga mat. Make sure you have space to move around. Wear comfortable clothing and take off your shoes and socks. Keep your CBD topical by your side.

2. Close your eyes and begin a series of deep inhales and exhales. Wiggle your feet. Are they sore from walking? Sometimes you get so used to aches and pains that you don't even notice them. Rub CBD topical between your hands and begin massaging your feet, your toes, and the arches of your feet.

3. Move up to your calves. Do they ache? What about the joints around your knees? Apply topical to reduce pain and inflammation to every part of your body that needs it. Work all the way up to your temples.

4. Reflect on your independence. Paying for massages is luxurious, and having a friend or partner give you one can make you feel loved. But you don't need anyone other than yourself for self-care.

Create a Friend Support Group

How does it help?

Friends provide valuable honest feedback, help you make smarter choices in your professional and personal life, and remind you that you're not alone. Integrate CBD into teas, tinctures, and treats during your social self-care time with your friends, and allow this phytocannabinoid to help you relax and share when you get together.

How to:

1. Suggest a monthly dinner party for your friends with the intention of providing support to one another. Pick a fun name that's fitting.
2. When you get together, agree that what happens at your friend support group stays in your friend support group. Everything said remains confidential.
3. Rotate where you meet so there's a different host each month. The host is responsible for making sure food and CBD are present for those who want it.
4. Go around in a circle and share how you're doing. Listen, relate, and offer advice when solicited. Most importantly, have fun!

Moisturize with CBD Hand Salve

How does it help?

The delicate skin on the hands is prone to dryness and premature aging. Practice self-care by keeping your hands moisturized and protected with CBD hand salve (available online and at health and beauty stores). CBD contains antioxidants, so the salve can heal your hands from the inside out.

How to:

1. Scoop out a dollop of CBD hand salve and begin to massage it onto your wrists.
2. Using your thumbs, rub the moisturizer into the palms of your hands, giving extra attention to areas that contain stress or discomfort.
3. Move along to your fingers. Enter full self-care mode by massaging the salve into one finger at a time, starting at the base and working all the way up to the tip. Take your time while doing this ritual, being sure to focus solely on how you're taking care of yourself.
4. Sit with your moisturized hands for about 5 minutes before moving on to another activity, to let your skin absorb the salve.

Call a Family Member

How does it help?
Connecting with a family member makes you feel loved and connected while offering them the same. But reaching out to family, especially if it's been a while, can be nerve-racking. CBD can ease your nerves and help you do things that scare you, even if they are the right move.

How to:
1. Eat CBD and wait for its effects to take hold.
2. You have control. Tell yourself that the conversation is going to go well, and you will be thankful for it. Go in with a positive attitude.
3. Call them! If it feels awkward, ask questions and let them do the talking. Actively listen and engage.
4. When they ask about you, share and be honest, but also honor your boundaries. You never need to tell your family everything.
5. Consider setting up a monthly or weekly time to catch up, so in the future, you avoid awkward stretches without communication. If the call went terribly, you never have to do it again. If it went well, reflect on how much better you feel for making the call, and appreciate the self-care.

Make a Gratitude List

How does it help?

CBD helps you open your heart and feel grateful by reducing irritating thoughts that may keep you stuck in a pattern of negativity. Capture those warm feelings by taking the time to make a gratitude list and appreciate how great your life really is.

How to:

1. Consume CBD to enter a state of mindfulness. With an open mind, observe your thoughts. How many of them are negative? Your thoughts shape your reality, which means that figuring out what's beautiful in your life produces tangible results. Take out a piece of paper and write "Gratitude List" across the top.

2. Make a list of things you are thankful for. They can be as small as your favorite cereal, or as big as freedom of speech. Don't forget to add self-care to the list! Once you start you will be stunned at how much there is to be grateful for.

3. To level up your gratitude lists and hold yourself accountable, create a gratitude email chain with friends. Their lists will inspire you and vice versa.

Try a Tarot Reading

How does it help?

Tarot cards are amazing self-reflection tools. Each card can offer insight into a situation, provide a screenshot of your current emotional state, and give you tips on how to proceed. Whether you're new to tarot or an experienced practitioner, what the cards reveal can be striking. Open your heart and mind with CBD, and settle into a calm and meditative state where you are ready to listen to what the cards have to say.

How to:

1. Pick up a pack of tarot cards if you don't already have some. For your first set, go for the Rider-Waite deck, because most tarot books reference it and the imagery is useful to learn. Each deck comes with a reference pamphlet, so don't stress if you don't know the card meanings. You will learn with practice.

2. Shuffle the deck while thinking about a question. Pull a card. Look its meaning up, but also use your intuition. Hold the card meditatively. What does it say to you?

continued on next page

3. Pulling cards can be nerve-racking. What if they say something negative? Take some CBD and simply observe what the cards say. Remember, there are no "bad" cards; each one offers important insight. It's your job to relax and read tarot from a receptive state.

4. Try another reading by laying out 3 cards in a row. Often, such a spread refers to the past, present, and future about a situation. They can help you look inward and be honest about what work you need to do to remedy a situation, or how to move a relationship to the next level.

Meditate under Blue Lighting

How does it help?

Spending time under blue lights has been shown to improve mood, so practice some mental self-care and swap out any harsh overhead bulbs with blue ones. CBD also has a positive effect on serotonin in the brain and gets rid of the blues, so you'll be in for some powerful CBD self-care that will help boost your mood.

How to:

1. Pick up and install some color-changing LED light bulbs, then place a dose of CBD under your tongue.
2. Make all the lights blue and sit with your CBD for at least 10 minutes, soaking in the mood-boosting hue.
3. If you're up for it, try doing some stretching and yoga moves in your blue light. Relax here for as long as you want. This time is yours for self-care, so do whatever makes you feel good.
4. Return to your CBD-enhanced blue meditation whenever you need to improve your mood and practice mental self-care.

Have a Heart-to-Heart

How does it help?

Having a serious talk with someone you love can be intimidating. However, when you don't, issues build up and become bigger than they need to be. Before you head into a heart-to-heart, take CBD to invite in calm compassion and focus.

How to:

1. Ingest some CBD. Remember that having this tough conversation wouldn't be difficult if you didn't care about the person you're talking to. Ground yourself in the love. Explain how you feel in concise, affirming "I" sentences ("I want to spend more time together" rather than "You don't spend enough time with me").
2. Be ready to listen and be flexible. If you rehearse the entire conversation ahead of time, you leave no room for unexpected opinions. Remember, if the goal is to work this out, you have to be ready to compromise.
3. End the conversation with a plan. The goal is to find a way toward mutually beneficial change. Revel in the feeling of accomplishment and emotional maturity for calmly tackling a tricky situation with love.

Be Selfish

How does it help?

Being selfish gets a bad rap, but when you neglect yourself, there is no way that you can hold it together for those around you. When you prioritize others so often, it may feel funny to put yourself first, but you can get over this mental block to self-care with invigorating CBD.

How to:

1. You have been giving others far too much of your time and mental space. Now it's time to focus on you. Start practicing self-care by placing a dose of CBD under your tongue.
2. Ask yourself if there is something you are not doing that you wish you were. If you feel this way, stop making others a priority over yourself. Politely tell those around you that you have somewhere else to be, then go do whatever it is that you want to do.
3. Continue to prioritize yourself and notice how much more you accomplish when you do.

Make CBD Lemonade

How does it help?

Making lemonade is an act of mindfulness that helps ground and center you. When life gives you lemons, make CBD lemonade. Turn worries into a stress-busting refreshing drink rich in vitamin C with this CBD recipe.

You will need:

1¾ cups sugar, 1 cup water, 1½ cups lemon juice, 1,000 milligrams CBD tincture

How to:

1. In a small saucepan, combine sugar and water. Bring the mixture to a boil. Stir frequently until sugar is dissolved. Allow the mixture to cool to room temperature. Cover and refrigerate until chilled.

2. In a pitcher, stir together lemon juice and sugar water. Add CBD tincture. Then add some ice cubes to a glass, pour yourself a serving of CBD lemonade, and literally chill. This recipe makes 4 servings, so share with friends or family who could also benefit.

Learn Your Love Language

How does it help?

Communicating with someone you love isn't always easy because you may have a different love language than your partner. There five love languages, or ways to express love: affirming words, acts of service, gifts, time, and touch. Concentrate with CBD to learn your and your partner's love languages. This will enhance the communication in your relationship and make you feel more fulfilled.

How to:

1. If you're not sure what your love language is, ingest a low dose of CBD to help you concentrate, then ask yourself, how do you express love? Are you a gift-giver? What makes you feel the most loved yourself? Is it physical touch from your partner?

2. Ask your partner what makes them feel loved. Do they have a specific memory or date that sticks out? If so, what about that moment was so exceptional?

3. Use a journal to take some notes about your love language, then share the information with your partner. Once you know both your and your partner's love languages, communication and expressions of love will become easier. Watch your relationship thrive as a result.

Practice Mindfulness

How does it help?

Mindfulness is the act of staying present in the moment. The immense self-care and health benefits of mindfulness include stress relief, treating heart disease, treating gastrointestinal issues, lowering blood pressure, reducing chronic pain, and improving sleep. CBD makes mindfulness easier by focusing the mind and quieting anxious thoughts to help keep you in the present, and it also shares some of the same benefits.

How to:

1. Squeeze a dose of CBD tincture under your tongue. Feel the texture. Taste the earthy and pungent notes. Inhale the woody scent up your nostrils.
2. Sit quietly. Take note of background noises, such as family talking or a radio in the background. Maybe it's raining outside.
3. Pick a color to count. For example, if you choose blue, you will look around your surroundings and make note of every blue thing you see. Color counting is a useful mindfulness tool to help root you in the present.
4. Keep electronics off. Just be here in the now. As the minutes pass, become mindful to how the CBD is relaxing you. Enjoy it and embrace these moments of self-care.

Watch Shooting Stars

How does it help?

Shooting stars can help remind you that you are part of a vast and miraculous world. Consuming CBD helps provide clarity and insight into the magical nature of the universe. Combine the two to remember that you are part of something greater, and that your time on this beautiful planet is limited and precious.

How to:

1. If you want, you can search for meteor shower calendars online to find the most starry night possible. Or just grab a blanket and your CBD and head somewhere with a clear view of the sky. Keep in mind that the sky is darkest during a new moon, which makes those nights the best for stargazing.
2. Take some CBD to ensure the plant-fueled serenity hits you in time for the show.
3. Lie back and enjoy. Make a wish for each star that you see. Try to find constellations and name planets. When life feels dull or boring, remember that you are part of this magnificent universe. Hard times fade, just like the seasons of the earth rotating around the sun.

Protect Your Skin

How does it help?

Sun exposure can lead to skin cancer, premature aging, and sunburns. Practice self-care and protect yourself by applying a CBD sunscreen with 30 SPF or higher. Your skin contains an abundance of cannabinoid receptors, the sites where CBD binds and gets to work, and research suggests that CBD regulates the renewal of skin cells and boosts the benefits of sunscreen.

How to:

1. Find a CBD sunscreen made by a brand you support.
2. Apply sunscreen 20 minutes before leaving your home. Be sure to apply it on your face and neck, but don't forget your ears and hands. Hands are often forgotten but are quick to show signs of aging.
3. If you're outside a lot, reapply every 2 hours. Self-care is removing worries, such as the negative effects of sun exposure, so you can have fun without fretting.

Forgive Someone

How does it help?

Forgiving someone who has hurt you may seem unfathomable, but research shows forgiveness can lower your stress levels. It's tough to forgive when you feel you've been wronged, but CBD can take the edge off difficult emotions and help you cultivate compassion. Have some CBD. Once you feel calm, ask yourself why you are holding on to anger. Does the anger feel good? Do you feel superior?

How to:

1. Remember that forgiveness doesn't mean forgetting, or that the conversation is over. It does mean that you're no longer giving the person or situation that wronged you all your power.
2. Take a moment to fully feel your anger. What did the incident teach you?
3. Then consider the other person, all their flaws, and why they mean so much to you. Can you trust them? Is your life happier with them in it?
4. Accept that the other person messed up. Embrace that you still want them in your life, or release them with goodwill. Reflect on how faulty human nature is, and even the ways you messed up in the past. Honor your decision to let it go by actively doing so.

Be Vain

How does it help?

Vanity is policed and frowned upon, but you deserve to pump yourself up and look your best. Boost your self-esteem with anxiety-busting CBD and then make yourself look as great as you can.

How to:

1. Eat some CBD and meditate on the benefits of welcoming vanity into your life. It's not always a bad thing. There's nothing wrong with wanting to look nice.

2. CBD's calming effects may help produce a creative mindset. Use your imagination to reflect on what looking nice means to you. For some, it's Hollywood glamour. For others, it's a natural look. Make a mood board to help capture inspiration.

3. If you're in need of new wellness products, consider shopping for those with CBD. Because CBD is an anti-inflammatory and antioxidant, it's found in face lotions, eye creams, and bath bombs.

4. Spend as much time as you need on your appearance. Don't let anyone make you feel bad for being vain. Decide that you only accept compliments. You're going to get a lot of them!

Say Less

How does it help?

Rather than ramble on in an argument, practice self-care by being up-front and just telling someone that you're upset. Sometimes the less you say, the better, because you get straight to the point, communicate clearly and rationally, and save yourself from letting your emotions take control. Boost your confidence and reduce fear with CBD and then express yourself grandly by saying less.

How to:

1. Take CBD to relax, then sit down with your feet planted on the floor. Take a cycle of breaths in and out to help facilitate a calm headspace.
2. When the conversation begins, practice active listening. Do not interrupt the other person. Hold space for both your opinions.
3. When it's your turn to speak, take your time. Boil your point down to one sentence. Rather than, "I can't believe that you were late again, you know how stretched thin I am, this is just like you..." assertively state: "I'd like you to respect my time."
4. Notice how much better you get your point across. Continue to be concise in your conversations.

Plan a Trip

How does it help?

Going away on vacation has been shown to decrease stress levels, and the more you plan the trip ahead, the less likely you are to be stressed while you're there. Use CBD to help you focus on planning a vacation and then go on it.

How to:

1. Consume a small dose of CBD to help you focus on planning.
2. Decide where you want to go. It can be a foreign country or to see family.
3. Find a time you can go. If needed, check in with bosses and ask for time off.
4. Pick a budget. Find affordable flights and hotels or home rentals.
5. Book away!
6. When you are able to get away and take the trip, everything will be neatly in order. All you have to do is get on board and have fun.

Stop Feeling Guilty

How does it help?
While guilt can be a chance to learn from the past and improve yourself, it is often unwarranted. Follow this ritual to let go of guilt with the serotonin-boosting effects of CBD. Once you stop feeling guilty, you can observe your choices from a rational point of view and use them as learning opportunities rather than a means of self-punishment.

How to:
1. Treat yourself to some CBD. Relax as the calming effects flood through your body. Why do you feel so guilty? Take out your journal and start writing. It's easier to see the truth when you look at it on paper and get out of your head.
2. If you messed up, apologize and make amends. Write down ways that you can improve your relationships moving forward without guilt. Self-soothe with CBD.
3. Practice self-care by owning your choices. You can't change the past. You did your best with what you had at the time. Let that guilt go.

Embrace CBD Face Oil

How does it help?

Face oil locks in your moisturizer, protecting your skin, and is an expert addition to any skin-based self-care routine. CBD enhances your face oil with its anti-inflammatory properties, which work to fight both breakouts and signs of aging.

How to:

1. Take your favorite face oil and add a few drops of coconut oil–based CBD tincture into the bottle.
2. Cleanse your skin. Gently scrub any dirt, debris, or makeup out of your pores.
3. Use a toner or astringent to tighten pores. Avoid anything alcohol-based if you have dry skin.
4. Apply your moisturizer or night cream, then apply your CBD-enhanced face oil.
5. Look at yourself in the mirror and feel good knowing that you've taken the time to do something nice for yourself—and know that your CBD face oil is helping you put your best face out there for the world to see.

Be Assertive

How does it help?
Being assertive allows you to stand up for what you want without being a bully or passive-aggressive. It's a powerful communication tactic in both professional and personal settings. Practicing this self-care exercise requires a calm and confident approach, which CBD can help with.

How to:
1. Assertiveness is most effective when you're calm and collected. Before trying out your skills, consume some CBD to bypass anxiety.
2. Remember to listen to the other party. Agree to disagree. There is not always one right answer. It's okay to have different opinions. Be patient (CBD can help with this too).
3. Assertiveness uses active problem solving, so be sure to offer concrete solutions to a problem. For instance, tell your boss that you cannot move your doctor's appointment, but you will complete your project afterward, and it will be awesome. You will feel confidence grow from being honest and assertive as you set clear boundaries and stick to them rather than let someone walk all over your time.

Connect with Your Spirit Guides

How does it help?

Many believe that we all have spirit guides that walk with us, from owls to dragons to superheroes. Follow this meditation to find yours as a source of strength to tap in to during tough times. If you're skeptical about the idea of spirit guides, just think of this as a fun, confidence-boosting exercise. Maybe you're more confident with a giant owl who follows you around and stares down enemies. Use CBD to sink into the moment and open up your mind, and this self-care exercise to exert your strength.

How to:

1. Sit on a yoga mat or pillow. Consume CBD tincture. Close your eyes and picture the following scenario. You are in a forest looking at a clearing at dusk. All is quiet except for the sound of nature.

2. As you step into the clearing you notice the glow of a fire. It's bright blue and purple with dancing yellow and orange flames. Its warmth feels comforting, powerful, and magnificent.

3. You sit down in front of the fire. You're meeting someone—an old friend. Slowly, out of the flames, your spirit guide emerges. It could be a majestic cat or even your grandmother. They sit down next to you. You feel completely safe and powerful in their presence.

4. Dusk begins to fade into night. You look up at the starry night and know that it's time to come home. Simply open your eyes to leave the clearing. There is no need to say goodbye to your guide. They are always with you. Whenever you feel scared, imagine your spirit guide and know that you have a powerful force within you to conquer your fears and help you get what you want.

Create a Mental Library

How does it help?

Unresolved worries can keep you up at night, creating even more woes from lack of sleep. Instead of worrying, create a mental library to file away your unwanted thoughts. CBD can help enhance this self-care exercise by helping you relax, stop worrying, and get a good night's sleep.

How to:

1. Take CBD, then envision your perfect library. Is it small and cozy? Is it a massive room in a mansion behind a secret doorway? There are no limits.

2. Your library exists in your mind. It's yours, and everything you store there is safe and preserved. When worries arise, file them away like books in your library. If the worry is important, you can come back and look into it later on. But for now, it's stored away. Your only job is to get a good night's rest.

3. When you've filed your worries away for the night, walk out of your library and lock the door behind you. Then close your eyes, appreciate the powerful effects of this CBD-driven self-care ritual, and drift off to sleep without those nighttime worries getting in the way.

Ride a Stationary Bike

How does it help?

Stationary bikes are a low-impact workout. This physical self-care exercise gives you the time to focus on how strong your body is, a thought that CBD can help enhance. Sometimes cardio can make your joints ache and become inflamed, but a CBD topical treats the pain before (and after) it starts, making your workout all about you.

How to:

1. Make a power playlist. Add any song that gets you amped up and ready to sweat.
2. Take some CBD then either go to a gym or hop on your home stationary bike and start riding. Begin on a low setting to get your blood pumping. Many stationary bikes have fun settings, such as hills or mountains, that make you feel like you're on an outdoor excursion rather than indoors. Enjoy the endorphins of cardio.
3. Ride for 30 minutes, or whatever length of time is best for you, then get off and stretch.
4. Rub CBD topical onto your joints to give them an extra dose of care.

Admire a Spiderweb

How does it help?

Gazing at the detailed handiwork of a spiderweb can help you appreciate the day-to-day beauty of the world around you, and will also help you be more present in the moment. That said, it's very normal to have a fear of spiders. But you don't want to miss out on the beautiful things in life just because you're afraid. Fortunately, CBD can help you relax and conquer your fear so you can take the time to admire something small but amazing.

How to:

1. Consume some CBD. As soon as you feel it starting to work, go hunting for spiderwebs!

2. When you find one don't knock it over or brush it away. Show some respect. Gaze into the web. Consider how much hard work went into creating this natural work of art. Remember that even on bad days, and even when everything feels ugly, there are entire other universes in the dusty corners around you.

3. If there is a spider on the web, don't worry. Quietly compliment the creature on its advantageous and lovely home.

Understand Another Perspective

How does it help?

If you and your friend or partner are arguing, taking the time to learn about their perspective can help you understand both that person and the world better. Relationships—and life—are more peaceful when everyone is getting along, but stepping out of your comfort zone can be scary. Use CBD to calm your nerves, cozy up to your partner or friend, and submerge yourself in love.

How to:

1. Take CBD to calm your nerves. So, you and someone you love have differing opinions. There's conflict as a result, but it's unnecessary. Think about how your backgrounds, upbringing, and life experience differ, and how that factors into your perspectives.

2. Realize that you can have hard conversations without it affecting your relationship. Keep it about the issue. Ask your person to explain their position. Actively listen.

3. Understanding where someone else is coming from doesn't mean you have to agree with them. You can keep your stance. But remember that it's okay to agree to disagree. The world is not black or white. It's okay to be open-minded and see the world through someone else's eyes.

Learn a New Language

How does it help?

Learning a new language is useful self-care that keeps your mind sharp and builds your compassion for other cultures. You'll improve your memory, stimulate creativity, and boost your multitasking abilities. You'll also learn about a new culture and appreciate those who are different from you. CBD can calm your mind and help you pay attention, making this self-care exercise easier and more fun.

How to:

1. Pick which language you want to learn, then consume a small dose of CBD to sharpen your focus. Select a language-learning method. Download apps or try online or in-person tutoring. Remember to have fun. This is something for you.

2. Set realistic goals, such as 30 new vocabulary words a week. Try flashcards (analog or electronic) to practice daily. Focus on short-term goals rather than long-term ones. Pick vocabulary topics that are important to you, such as traveling, shopping, or dining.

3. Show off your skills! Practice makes perfect, and it's fun to celebrate your successes with others.

Take an Apology Break

How does it help?

Saying "I'm sorry" can turn into a reflex. Maybe you apologize when you don't need to and, as a result, shoulder blame you're not responsible for. With the aid of CBD for clarity, calm, focus, and mindfulness, practice self-care by taking back your power with an apology break.

How to:

1. Begin each day by meditating for 10 minutes after consuming CBD. If you prefer CBD at night, meditate before bed. The goal of your meditation is to become aware of saying "I'm sorry." Sometimes you may say "I'm sorry," but what you really mean is "I don't want to fight," "I'm hurt," or "I need love." Use CBD to lower your stress levels and tune in to what you really need (and the courage to ask for it).

2. Throughout the day, watch how often you apologize. If you mess up at work or are mean to your partner, an apology is warranted. But if you turn down social obligations due to a work deadline, or for much-needed self-care, an apology is not warranted. Just like an apology is not needed when someone bumps into you on the sidewalk or your pharmacist is taking so long to serve you that a line forms behind you. These are not your fault.

continued on next page

3. Learn the difference between small things that inconvenience others and intentional acts that cause harm.

4. The next time you want to say "I'm sorry," try "Thank you" instead. For instance, if you're slightly late handing in a work assignment due to a family emergency, rather than apologize for something out of your control, say "Thank you for your understanding, I appreciate it." When you flip the script to a positive narration rather than one of blame, others follow your lead.

Practice the Law of Attraction

How does it help?

The Law of Attraction states that when you think positively, you attract positivity to your life. When you think negatively, you attract negativity to your life instead. CBD helps remove worries that keep you stuck in negative thinking patterns, leading you toward a positive mindset associated with a longer lifespan and a more productive life. Paired with CBD, which lowers worries, believing you can do it helps you achieve it.

How to:

1. Using a pen and paper, write out all your worries and fears. Then tear it up and throw it away.

2. Consume some CBD. As it takes effect, write down a new list of everything that you want to gain or achieve. It can be a new job, a certain amount of money in your bank account, a dream vacation, or literally anything you want. Hang it up somewhere you can see it.

3. Then begin each day by mentally listing your achievements, everything from career advances to surviving a horrible breakup, to remind yourself how strong you are. Keep CBD on you and take it as needed to help fight off negative thinking.

Learn All the Words to a Song

How does it help?

Learn all the words to your favorite song so that you have a karaoke go-to. Or maybe you just need to belt out some ballads around the house. CBD can clear your mind to help you focus and memorize all the lyrics so you can hurry up and get to the fun part—singing an entire song in the shower or at karaoke with friends.

How to:

1. Look up the lyrics to your favorite song and listen to the tune repeatedly with the goal of understanding the meaning. It's easier to get into a song if you connect emotionally with the lyrics.
2. Practice. Sing out loud while you do the dishes, in the shower, while you drive to work. If you ever feel shy about singing, ease your nerves with some CBD.
3. Break out the song at karaoke, or at the house when you need a burst of fun just for you.

Meditate with Rose Quartz

How does it help?

Crystal healers say that rose quartz helps promote healing, self-love, and personal fulfillment, and CBD can help you open your heart and mind to all possibilities. Meditate with rose quartz to practice self-love with an open, CBD-powered mind.

How to:

1. Obtain some rose quartz. The pretty crystal is said to open the heart chakra, an area over the chest associated with self-love, compassion, and healing.
2. Sit cross-legged on the floor or on a yoga mat. Drop a dose of CBD tincture under your tongue. As it dissolves, hold the rose quartz in your palm. Inhale for 4 counts; exhale for 4 counts. Repeat this breath pattern until you feel calm.
3. Press the rose quartz right to your heart. Imagine it removing self-doubt. Repeat a mantra in your head, such as "I am loved" or simply "I am okay." Visualize the pink stone soaking into your chest and healing any hurt. You are loved, and you are okay. Repeat this self-care ritual whenever you need a hug.

Support a Local Candidate

How does it help?

Better understand your local politics by researching neighborhood politicians and helping one who speaks to you. Supporting a candidate is rewarding work that helps you feel involved in your community, but it can be trying at times. Keep CBD around for when your mind needs a reboot.

How to:

1. Find a local candidate who inspires you. Look up your district's US representative, or go smaller. If you don't know where to start, look up an issue that's important to you, which can be as big as gender equality or as local as land use in your hometown.

2. Contact the campaign to see how you can help. For some people, donating money is easy, but local candidates also need people to help make phone calls, go door to door, or help them in others ways that require more time and attention.

3. Politics are stressful, so before you sign up to volunteer, take some CBD and use it to self-soothe as needed. Then go out and tell your friends about a candidate who inspires you, and feel empowered to help someone you believe in.

Take a Nap

How does it help?
Naps increase your cognitive function, creativity, and productivity—and taking one can be an ultimate form of self-care—but sometimes it can be hard to turn your brain off. CBD, in any form, will help you fall asleep and stay asleep, so use this calming cannabinoid to get into rest mode.

How to:
1. Put a dose of CBD tincture under your tongue.
2. If you must wake up at a certain time, set an alarm, but nothing too abrupt.
3. Snuggle up on your couch or bed and remind yourself that rest is important, and it's okay to take care of yourself by getting the sleep you need. Let the CBD wash away your worries, then help you drift off to a productive, restful slumber.

Give Out Care Kits for the Homeless

How does it help?

Helping others promotes a sense of purpose, lowers blood pressure, may help with chronic pain, and just feels good, so practice self-care by making an easy care kit to give to homeless people as you walk by. It's okay to feel sad about the injustice after interacting with people, so make sure to care for yourself by keeping CBD on hand.

How to:

1. Collect basic necessities such as tampons, socks, snacks, gloves, and lip balm. Pack them into small bags that you can carry with you.

2. When walking around, if you pass a homeless person, hand them a care kit. Make eye contact. Chat for a minute. One of the most degrading parts about being homeless is feeling invisible.

3. Seeing people suffer can be tough, and you may feel guilty for having what you do when others don't have much. Self-soothe with CBD so you have the energy to open your heart and keep on giving.

Make a Bucket List

How does it help?

When you write down your goals they become easier to accomplish, so practice self-care by making a bucket list to check your goals off one by one as you achieve them. Your bucket list will keep you motivated and excited about the future, and it can help you feel creative as you brainstorm all your future achievements. CBD can relieve stress if your goals feel overwhelming.

How to:

1. Take a strong dose of CBD to get rid of any doubts or negativity, then take out your pen and paper and write down what you want out of life. It can be a marriage, money, a job, a pet, a vacation, or more confidence. These are your goals.
2. Hang up the list somewhere you can see.
3. Let your list haunt you a little bit. When you set goals, they can nag at you—use this motivation to get them done.
4. Each time you complete a goal (and you will!), cross it off and celebrate your accomplishments.

Try a Banana Smoothie

How does it help?
Think of CBD as a nutritional supplement in a delicious and healthy CBD-infused smoothie. Studies indicate that CBD stimulates metabolism through the binding of cannabinoid receptors, which will make you feel healthy and nourished after you try this drink.

You will need:
2 peeled and sliced bananas, ½ cup peanut butter, 2 cups vanilla almond milk, 1 tablespoon honey, 30 milligrams CBD tincture

How to:
1. Add all the ingredients to a blender. Pulse a few times to chop up all the ingredients and then blend on high until smooth, about 30 seconds or until the ingredients are well combined.
2. Pour your smoothie into a cup. Sip it slowly. Enjoy not only the delicious taste but the knowledge that you're taking care of your body by filling it with protein, potassium, calcium, and fiber.

Do a Body Scan for Mental Self-Care

How does it help?

You may find yourself so trapped inside your own head that you don't even realize how stressed out you are! A body scan is a perfect mental self-care exercise that can help you identify where you're holding on to worry and tension—and let it go. Use a CBD capsule or tincture to get rid of worries that keep you out of touch with your body. Afterward, a CBD topical can address pain directly to areas of the body that are holding tension.

How to:

1. Sit down on your yoga mat with your CBD tincture. Drop some under your tongue. Complete a few cycles of breaths as the CBD dissolves.
2. Take a look inside your head. Notice your worries as an impartial observer. Talk to yourself with the same kind honesty that you'd give a friend.
3. Now move down to your chest. Does it feel like an elephant is sitting on your chest or your heart is going to explode? In this case, it's unlikely that you're having a heart attack, and there is no elephant in the room. You're just stressed out.

continued on next page

4. Now that you're aware of your stress levels, sit and take deep breaths in and out. Stay calm and try to bring in perspective.

5. Often, action is the best way to combat anxiety. If you're worried about work, get up and get to it. If you're worried about a romantic partner, reach out and remind them how much you love them. And don't forget about you! First and foremost, tell yourself how much you love yourself. That's what self-care is all about.

Escape with Nature Sounds

How does it help?

Listening to nature sounds helps you relax, stay mindful (in the present moment), and sleep better. CBD helps you sink into relaxation, and white noise calms worrisome thoughts.

How to:

1. Download a white noise app, then drop a relaxing dose of CBD under your tongue and choose your preferred nature sound.
2. Close your eyes. Feel the hemp plant fill your mouth, and melt into tranquility. Breathe with the sound of the rain, or whichever nature sound you have on.
3. Fully release yourself to the sound you're playing. Let go of all your worries as you engulf yourself in the sound of waves, rain, or a forest. When you're ready to come back to the world, gently open your eyes and turn off the white noise. Carry the peaceful feeling that this self-care ritual has given you, and take comfort in knowing that this type of mental/spiritual self-care is easily accessible whenever you need it.

Turn Off Your Phone

How does it help?

Phones are stressful little noisemakers that demand a lot of your attention. Practice self-care by just turning your phone off! Use CBD to help yourself be fully present in the moment. The relaxing properties of CBD help quell work worries and the habit of checking social media, allowing you to focus purely on self-care.

How to:

1. Have some CBD, then, once the calm sets in, turn off your phone for 1 hour. Enjoy the silence or pick an activity to become fully engulfed in. When you enter "the zone" while rock climbing, playing music, or dancing with someone you love, it's known as "flow state." Nothing else matters but the present moment.

2. Whether you're engaged in self-care rituals, work, or chores around the house, notice how productive you are with your phone off. You begin to value your time more. Your stress levels lower and you sleep better.

3. Try to turn off your phone (or put it on airplane mode) for a little bit each week. Start small and work up to a level you are comfortable with.

Make and Use Affirmation Stones

How does it help?
CBD can calm you down, but an affirmation stone—a stone with an uplifting message on it—carried in your pocket or held during a meditation can help direct your attention toward a goal. For example, if your stone says "I am loved," you can meditate about how much love is in your life. Making an affirmation stone is also a calming craft activity; taking a low dose of CBD before you begin can help you focus as you create.

How to:
1. Pick up some flat stones, acrylic paint or a metallic permanent marker, and some brushes from your local craft store.
2. Prepare an area in which to work (it may get messy), then take a low dose of CBD.
3. Pick an affirmation special to you, such as "I am worthy of love" or "Stay strong." Paint or write it on your stone. Set it aside until it's dry.
4. Place the stone in your pocket or purse. Take it out and read it whenever you need to take a moment to close your eyes and practice self-care.

See Someone's Good Side

How does it help?

Stop wasting energy on people you're in conflict with by taking a moment to try to understand them. Use CBD to get over the initial hump of being the bigger person and showing compassion toward someone you don't like. Because the cannabinoid calms you down, it lowers ego-based hesitation to give someone a second chance.

How to:

1. Consume a dose of CBD to feel more comfortable and compassionate.
2. Visualize a person that you're not fond of. Then use a beginner's mind, which means approaching things from a fresh, open, and curious perspective, to mentally say nice things, such as that you appreciate their work ethic or personal style.
3. Eventually you'll begin to feel softer toward this person. If you see them face-to-face, offer the same compassion. It will free you from the prison of hating them. Your obsession with them will also dwindle, and eventually you won't even think of them much.

Try CBD Eye Cream

How does it help?

The skin around your eyes is extremely sensitive. Fortunately, CBD's anti-inflammatory properties help soothe the delicate skin around your eyes to combat the puffiness and dryness that lead to wrinkles. By pairing CBD with the use of an eye cream you take time just for you to pat away the stress of the day.

How to:

1. Wash your face with warm water using your favorite cleanser. Make circular motions with your fingers to wash away the debris of the day. After you rinse your face, apply your favorite moisturizer to your face.
2. Scoop out an appropriate amount of your favorite eye cream. Add 1 drop CBD oil. Gentle combine them using your finger and the palm of your hand.
3. Carefully apply your enhanced eye cream to the delicate skin around your eyes.
4. Sip a cup of tea and relax as your nourishing eye cream soaks into your skin. If you want a stress-relieving boost of CBD, squirt a dose of tincture into your tea. Appreciate the time you were able to set aside to prioritize yourself.

Further Resources

How to Safely Source CBD

CBD is very popular right now. Everyone wants a taste of the cannabinoid. But while it's terrific news that so many people have access to CBD, this also means that scammers are trying to make a quick buck by selling low-quality products. Since CBD is still largely unregulated, a lot of companies are doing whatever they can to cash in, including selling products that contain unsafe additives or even pesticides. This means that before you can incorporate CBD into your self-care routine, you need to make sure you're doing whatever you can to purchase safe, clean, high-quality CBD products.

Shop with Reputable Retailers

The first way to make sure you're purchasing high-quality CBD is to shop with reputable retailers. If you live in a US state where cannabis is legal, you can obtain trustworthy CBD products at a dispensary. In legal states, in addition to hemp-derived CBD, dispensaries also sell CBD extracted from marijuana with a low THC ratio. Remember that anything hemp-based must have THC levels below 0.3 percent. Even in US medical states, where CBD and cannabis are available with a medical card, most dispensaries sell dependable CBD products that anyone can purchase. If you don't want to shop at a dispensary, try your local CBD store. You can also legally buy hemp-derived CBD online. Websites such as www.leafly.com review CBD brands and can offer insight from other consumers.

Read Labels

They say not to judge a book by its cover, but you can learn a lot from reading the label of a CBD product. Make sure that the label states how much CBD the product contains, rather than merely the words *hemp oil*. Hemp oil can simply mean oil from hemp seeds, which contains trace amounts of CBD, but not enough to justify selling it as a CBD product.

It's also useful to know how the CBD is extracted from the plant. Do not use anything made with toxic solvents such as butane, hexane, and propane. Ethanol (grain alcohol) is a safe extraction method. Many companies use CO_2, which is also a reliable method.

You should also make sure your CBD's label clarifies whether it's full spectrum, broad spectrum, or CBD isolate. Remember that full spectrum keeps all the other plant goodness in addition to the CBD, broad spectrum includes some of the rest of the plant, and isolate is pure CBD. Different people prefer different extractions, but regardless of what you want to use, it's a good sign when a product clarifies what you're getting on the label. Check out some of the CBD companies in the following Resource List for happy, healthy shopping.

Resource List

Online Connections

CBD Choice
https://cbdchoice.com

Healthy Hemp Oil
www.healthyhempoil.com

CBD Outlet Online
www.cbdoutletonline.com

Healthy Hemp Outlet
www.hhoutlet.com

The CBD Store
www.thecbdstores.com

Lord Jones
https://lordjones.com

Discover CBD
www.discovercbd.com

Pure CBD Vapors
www.purecbdvapors.com

Elixinol
www.elixinol.com

Papa & Barkley
www.papaandbarkley.com

Foria
www.foriawellness.com

Plant People
https://plantpeople.co

Project CBD
www.projectCBD.org

Sunday Scaries
https://sundayscaries.com

TribeTokes
www.tribetokes.com

Vireo Health
https://vireohealth.com

Online Magazines

Consumer Reports
www.consumerreports.org

High Times
https://hightimes.com

Leafly
www.leafly.com

Lifehacker
https://lifehacker.com

Merry Jane
https://merryjane.com

Miss Grass
www.missgrass.com

Standard US/Metric Measurement Conversions

VOLUME CONVERSIONS	
US Volume Measure	**Metric Equivalent**
⅛ teaspoon	0.5 milliliter
¼ teaspoon	1 milliliter
½ teaspoon	2 milliliters
1 teaspoon	5 milliliters
½ tablespoon	7 milliliters
1 tablespoon (3 teaspoons)	15 milliliters
2 tablespoons (1 fluid ounce)	30 milliliters
¼ cup (4 tablespoons)	60 milliliters
⅓ cup	90 milliliters
½ cup (4 fluid ounces)	125 milliliters
⅔ cup	160 milliliters
¾ cup (6 fluid ounces)	180 milliliters
1 cup (16 tablespoons)	250 milliliters
WEIGHT CONVERSIONS	
US Weight Measure	**Metric Equivalent**
½ ounce	15 grams
1 ounce	30 grams
2 ounces	60 grams
¼ pound (4 ounces)	115 grams
½ pound (8 ounces)	225 grams
¾ pound (12 ounces)	340 grams
1 pound (16 ounces)	454 grams
OVEN TEMPERATURE CONVERSION	
350 degrees F	180 degrees C